A 30-Day Journey into Christian Yoga

Faith *with a* Twist

Hillary D. Raining & Amy Nobles Dolan

Photographs of the yoga poses by the authors were taken by Bill Ecklund, a portrait and fashion photographer who lives in Wayne, Pennsylvania. Visit his website, www.billecklund.com, to view more of his work.

Scripture quotations are from the New Revised Standard Version of the Bible, copyright © 1989 National Council of the Churches of Christ in the United States of America. Used by permission. All rights reserved.

Prayers from *Lesser Feasts and Fasts* © Domestic and Foreign Missionary Society are reprinted with gracious permission.

Psalm passages are from the Psalter in *The Book of Common Prayer*.

© 2018 Forward Movement
All rights reserved.
ISBN: 978-0-880-28456-1
Printed in USA

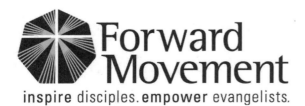

Forward Movement

inspire disciples. empower evangelists.

A 30-Day Journey into Christian Yoga

Faith *with a* Twist

Hillary D. Raining & Amy Nobles Dolan

Forward Movement
Cincinnati, Ohio

Table of Contents

A Word from the Authors

Come to me, all you that are weary and are carrying heavy burdens, and I will give you rest. Take my yoke upon you, and learn from me; for I am gentle and humble in heart, and you will find rest for your souls.
—Matthew 11:27-29

We live in an interesting time for organized religion. Judging by the current trends and data, more and more people identify with the "spiritual but not religious" label and have turned to contemplative practices like yoga to bring them into closer relationship with God. *Faith with a Twist: A 30-Day Journey into Christian Yoga* seeks to connect the spiritual and religious by blending the ancient wisdom of the church and the ancient spiritual practice of yoga.

Frequently, attempts to blend yoga and Christianity fail to do justice to both traditions—sacrificing the wisdom of one tradition for the other. In this way, each discipline tends to be watered down. Building upon our vocations as an Episcopal priest and a yoga teacher and trainer, we seek to weave the traditional eight limbs of yoga together with the church's understanding and emphasis on living a holy life. Our prayer is that this approach presents a unique blend of spiritual practices and religious wisdom that will encourage and nourish the body, mind, and soul of the yoga novice and the experienced practitioner alike. We have purposefully included both traditional poses and modified, chair-based poses because we believe yoga is a practice available to everyone, regardless of age or physical ability.

Connecting our deeply rooted Christian faith with our love of yoga, we have created this 30-day journey as a guide for those seeking to grow in their love of God. This book offers a different prayer, reflection, and practice for each day of a month-long journey. In addition to the core meditation material, we include ways to use this resource in different seasons of the church year—and different seasons of your lives. Yoga has deepened our faith, and we hope this book full of prayers, wisdom, and practices helps transform your spiritual life.

Namaste,
Hillary & Amy

Using this Resource

Most of us have a hard time with stillness. We would rather move—run, climb, dance, and prance. Our ancient yoga teachers knew this, so they devised *asana* practice as a moving prayer—a series of motions designed to draw our awareness inward. Yoga is movement to create stillness—physical stillness that we are able to sustain in *savasana* and mental stillness throughout our practice and into our days.

Being faithful to Jesus and practicing yoga can go hand in hand. This guide incorporates vital elements of Christianity (including several beloved prayers from the Episcopal tradition) and provides context and explanation around the ancient spiritual wisdom of yoga. Each daily meditation includes prayers, reflections, and practices that are designed to be used every day for a month. Ideally, you will carve out 15-30 minutes to pray, read and reflect upon a meditation and practice yoga poses. Each day also offers a bit of yoga insight and tips. We encourage you to move through all sixteen poses each day, at your own pace. The series of poses is featured in the special full-color section, from pages 50-81.

A key principle of yoga will be explored in-depth for three days. Three is a powerful number in both Christianity and yoga. For Christians, the number corresponds to many important biblical teachings, notably in the three persons of the Trinity—Father, Son, and Holy Spirit—and in the three days that Jesus spent in the tomb before his resurrection. As Christians, we are called to love the Lord our God with mind, body, and soul. In yoga, three areas of attention (known in Sanskrit as *tristhana*) are a part of every movement—the breath (*pranayama*), the gazing point (*dristhi*), and the posture itself (*asana*). These three elements work together to purify or cleanse the mind, body, and soul.

On the first day, the reflection is a little longer as the concept is explained in depth. On this day, a verse of yoga scripture or *sutra* is included. These verses are from a book called *The Yoga Sūtras of Patañjal (YS)*, written around 400 BCE and widely regarded as the foundational text of yoga. In addition to the original Sanskrit and literal translation, we have included our own understanding of each sutra. On the second day, we reflect on the same moral principle from a Christian perspective.

The third day is a little different. Both our Christian faith and our yoga practices have taught us that it is necessary and good to seek wisdom from scripture, authors, and experienced teachers. There is also another rich way to study: the "inner teacher." On the third day of each set of moral principles, we will tune into our inner teacher or to the Holy Spirit within. We have included open-ended prompts as an invitation to turn inward to reflect. This may include journaling or sitting in meditation, exploring how you personally understand, experience, and yearn to grow into each moral principle.

This workbook is perfect for individual use, group practice, or by religious communities looking to help members incorporate the principles and practice of yoga into their faith lives. Indeed, the month-long approach provides an excellent structure to this practice of blending faith and yoga. Thirty days is enough time to make (and break) a habit; we hope these thirty days can help you establish a habit that will support you for a lifetime.

We believe *Faith with a Twist* can enrich the most seasoned yoga practitioner and the yoga novice. The book is designed with adults in mind, but older youth and teens will enjoy this experiential way to pray. The book can also be a terrific resource for prayer groups, Bible and seasonal studies, and retreats. Participants should have their own copy of *Faith with a Twist* as a guide to which they return again and again.

The Appendix includes a glossary of terms as well as a guide for pronunciation. There are also suggestions on how to adapt these practices in other settings and seasons and a list of resources for additional study.

Although we perceive yoga as a spiritual practice and not exercise, it does require some physical exertion and movement. As with any new physical activity, you may wish to consult with a physician before you begin. If you are using a chair for the modified poses, we suggest selecting a sturdy one with arms. Make sure any cushion is firmly attached.

Sample Day

A typical *Faith with a Twist* session begins with a prayer, followed by a reflection and the setting of intentions, which leads directly into the physical postures and breath habits of the practice. Each session should end with a period of silence and total relaxation, allowing the Holy Spirit to refresh and refine you.

The lay-flat binding of the book allows you to place the resource on the ground near your mat or on a table. This enables you to easily follow the prayers, reflections, and poses each day.

Pray
Starting with prayer sets the tone for a practice that will stir your heart and soul. For the thirty-day period of this book, we have selected prayers from *Lesser Feasts and*

Fasts, *The Book of Common Prayer,* or other Episcopal prayer resources. You can also choose prayers that are particularly meaningful to you or your community. You may consider writing your own prayers, particularly as you embark on a second or third month of practice.

Reflect

These short reflections explore the moral principles of yoga and how faith guides our beliefs and responses. As we read and contemplate these meditations, we are asked to don a posture of humility and an openness to new paths.

The reflections invite you into a time of intention setting. Perhaps you are being called to give up something that might be distracting you from God or to take up a practice that will lead you into a deeper relationship. Perhaps you simply need to spend some time quietly digesting a new realization. Whatever your intentions, they will set the tone for your practice.

Practice

Using the special section as a guide, perform each of the postures slowly and with intention. Focus on your breathing. Be attentive to your body. Quiet your mind and open yourself to God.

Once you have finished practicing the active poses, you may be tempted to jump right back into your day. Instead, spend 10-15 minutes (as you are able) in *savasana*—corpse pose. Breathe comfortably and allow your experience to imprint itself in your mind and soul. Listen for the Holy Spirit in the rhythm of your breath, and be aware of the changes and new understandings you may discover in your body, mind, and soul. As you end, place your hands in prayer position over your heart and bow to your fellow students, teacher, and to God in thanksgiving for this time and growth and say "*Namaste*," which means "the divine in me honors the divine in you."

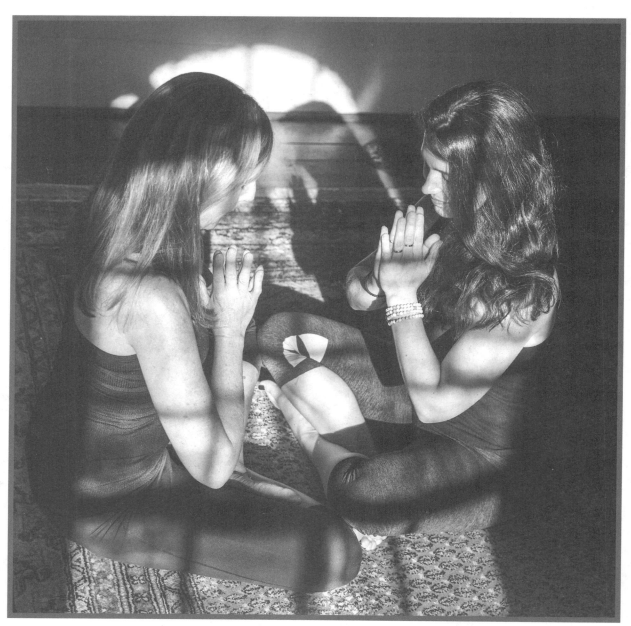

Authors Amy Nobles Dolan and Hillary D. Raining

Introduction

Do you not know that your body is a temple of the Holy Spirit within you, which you have from God, and that you are not your own? —1 Corinthians 6:19

In the United States, most people have been introduced to yoga through classes at health clubs and gyms. While it's wonderful these classes have brought yoga to so many, this method of introduction has framed the practice as merely (or primarily) exercise. Though yoga is great physical exercise, it is much more than that. The postures and principles that make up what we think of yoga were created as a spiritual practice some 3,000 years ago. Yoga is, at its deepest root, a spiritual practice, a tool to help people draw closer to God.

We are taught through our Christian faith to love God. Yoga teaches us to love ourselves as God's creation. For most of us, loving ourselves is much harder to do than loving God. Author and yoga leader Rolf Gates writes in his book, *Meditations from the Mat*, that a "spiritual practice is not about locking up all the unruly aspects of yourself, in the hope that they will never get free. Spiritual practice is about turning on the light—and the light is love."

The practice of yoga proposes to teach us to love all aspects of ourselves—not just the nice stuff that we're proud of but also the things we struggle with. We are to learn to love ourselves completely because God loves us completely. God doesn't love some perfected version of us that we might become one day. God loves us right here and right now—as we already are. Once we have embraced this fact (and, in doing so, have embraced ourselves), the next step is to love others even though they aren't perfect yet either.

As we lovingly accept one another for all that we are and all that we are not, we begin to live together as God intended. We begin to live into God's intention for this world. While we individual humans aren't perfect, love is. Through our love for ourselves and through our love for one another, we express the bit of God that abides in us. We allow that spark of God to shine through us in our lives.

This process isn't easy, and we need practices that can help guide us. Luckily, yoga traditions provide a wonderful structure to embrace and build our practice of loving God, ourselves, and others. Yoga offers a concise description of spiritual practice that includes two aspects: *abhyasa* (practice) and *vairagya* (renunciation). *Abhyasa* is the chance to practice habits and behaviors that we would like to develop in our real lives. Our yoga mats become laboratories where we test these things. Our mats are safe, contained places where we can experiment with how these habits and behaviors feel and with how hard or how surprisingly easy they are. Because we are practicing, it is, as a matter of course, okay to mess up. We just try again.

Vairagya (renunciation) focuses on taking what we practice or learn through yoga and applying it to our lives. Traditional definitions of *vairagya* can sound intimidating. They speak of shedding self-defeating behaviors; *vairagya* is seen as—to quote yoga master BKS Iyengar—"the elimination of all that hinders progress or refinement."

These explanations of renunciation can sound more daunting than inspiring, especially when we have become culturally conditioned to being overly critical or judgmental of one another and ourselves. The intention behind *vairagya* is not critical at all. Renunciation simply cannot be fully understood on its own—it needs to be unified with *abhyasa* (practice) to be accurately grasped. When we approach the two aspects of spiritual practice together, we are able to receive the deeper gifts of yoga.

There is no pressure or need to succeed—we have the freedom to practice all we want. The more we practice, the more these newly formed habits will become second nature. Almost before we realize it, we begin making the same changes on our mats and in our real lives. We come to shed self-defeating behaviors. We see obstacles to our progress more clearly and learn to gracefully navigate around them. That is simply the way yoga—and the wisdom of the Holy Spirit—works.

Once we start practicing (*abhyasa*) and assume the yoke of yoga, we will quickly discover the riches, comfort, and rest for our souls that our Christian spiritual practices offer in our daily lives. Once we experience those riches and comfort, continued commitment (*vairagya*) becomes easier, and we find that our burdens have become lighter.

As the well-known yoga teacher and Sanskrit scholar K. Pattabhi Jois said, "Practice, and all is coming."

The Foundations of a Spiritual Practice

I will show you what someone is like who comes to me, hears my words, and acts on them. That one is like a man building a house, who dug deeply and laid the foundation on rock; when a flood arose, the river burst against that house but could not shake it, because it had been well built. But the one who hears and does not act is like a man who built a house on the ground without a foundation. When the river burst against it, it fell, and great was the ruin of that house. —Luke 6:47-49

Every practice needs a foundation upon which to rest. This foundation supports and protects the practice. In any spiritual practice, yoga included, the foundation supports and protects the relationship we are developing with God.

Our time in *asana* (yoga postures) on our mats is the foundation for a healthy yoga practice. This can help us reinforce and—when needed—recreate the foundation of our spiritual practices. For some, a yoga practice and a Christian spiritual practice is one and the same. For others, a regular yoga practice is a wonderful model for how to construct a spiritual practice.

It is up to each of us to figure out what foundation we need to build in order to deepen our relationship with God. The critical point here is that we must make the choice and the commitment. Both intention and action are required on our part. The decision is totally personal. The choice is ours to make.

Once we make our decision and commitment, our practices can (and should) be open to change. Our practices should feel good. Our practices should fit into our lives. After all, at their fundamental (foundational!) level, our practices are manifestations of our relationship with God. While our relationship with God is always and forever present, the way it materializes in our lives changes over time. Our practices will ebb and flow in intensity with the twists and turns of our lives. The form our practices take is secondary. What is crucial is that we maintain commitment to our practice. That commitment is the rock on which the rest of our practice stands.

'ngs First: Show Up!

ı, take courage! Do not let your hands be weak,
work shall be rewarded. —2 Chronicles 15:7

Ĭo benefit from any kind of practice, we have to show up. To increase the likelihood that we will show up, we need to schedule the practice into our days. For our purposes, this means setting aside time on our calendar for yoga. Because yoga is a spiritual practice, we are, in essence, making an appointment and showing up to meet with God. Creating this "appointment time" means figuring out and committing to a routine that works for you—you may unroll your mat once a week on a Thursday night or every morning. For a practice to work, for a true commitment to a practice to form, the practice must be customized to the rhythms of your life. It doesn't matter how much you practice yoga but that you follow through with your commitment and appointment time with God.

Ch-ch-ch-Changes

For everything there is a season, and a time for every
matter under heaven... —Ecclesiastes 3:1

Yes, commitment is important, but we also must be flexible. Life is change, and nothing stays the same. If our practice becomes a burden when life veers in a new direction, we need to change it or we will eventually stop practicing, no matter how strong our will.

For our yoga practice, this means that on some days, we may only squeeze in 15 minutes on the mat, while on other days we will have plenty of time to move. And sometimes, we will flop down into *savasana* (resting pose at the end of practice) after dragging ourselves through a brief series of standing poses and call it a day.

The same is true with our prayer lives. Some days, we will have a rich and wonderful conversation with God, and on other days, we might feel disconnected and alone. Be open to changes both in how you pray and how you practice. There is no single right way for everyone at every time. While we recommend embracing different prayers and practices, we urge you to remain firm in your faithfulness to these principles. Committing to prayer and practice–even as they take different shapes and forms—provides strength and support for our everyday lives. There is a lot of grace and mercy in prayer and practice, and it all counts.

We Give, and We Receive

*The one who sows sparingly will also reap sparingly, and
the one who sows bountifully will also reap bountifully.*
—2 Corinthians 9:6

If we want to receive more benefits from our yoga practice, then we can increase
the energy and focus we pour into it. In Sanskrit, this is called *tapas*, which translates
as zeal. *Tapas* is the fire that drives us. In *asana* practice, we bring *tapas* to the mat,
but we also carry this zeal with us into the rest of our day. This should be true of any
spiritual practice, especially prayer.

The benefits we reap are the reason we return regularly to our practice. If what we're
doing in our spiritual practice feels like all work and no reward, then we need to re-
think it. We need to listen to ourselves and respect our needs. As long as our prayers
and practice come from our deepest hearts and are motivated by a desire to find
connection to God, we can (and should) trust them.

Climbing the Learning Curve

*May you be made strong with all the strength that comes
from his glorious power, and may you be prepared to
endure everything with patience.* —Colossians 1:11

Sometimes, the tools of our practice are hard to master at first. We have to devote serious
time and energy to climbing a learning curve before we can truly settle into the practice.

The same is true for most any discipline we undertake. At first, any new practice may
seem like hard work, but in time and with dedication it becomes natural and fits gracefully
into our lives. Once we start seeing the benefits and experiencing the rewards, it's easy to
stay motivated to stick with the practice. The initial period of learning is the toughest.

It helps to make a real commitment to try a new thing for a set (and reasonable)
length of time. Making a deliberate decision and finite commitment provides the time
and space to really experience a practice before you feel moved to judge it. With
thirty days of prayer, reflection, and practice, this book is designed to give you the
space and time to experience and discern whether it's the right method for you.

At the Root of It All, a Word

In the beginning was the Word, and the Word was with God, and the Word was God. —John 1:1

In nearly every yoga class, practice is closed with the word and gesture of *namaste*. One definition of *namaste* stands out as the perfect summation of what we are doing when we practice yoga. This definition is: "The God in me greets the God in you," or "The divine in me greets the divine in you." Here we are back at the foundation of our practice! We begin by seeking the divine within ourselves through our practice. We end up, having journeyed through our practice, recognizing the divine within us all.

Sometimes when you're pondering a broad topic, a single, small element beautifully encapsulates the spirit of the whole. In yoga, the greeting *namaste* does just this. Aadil Palkhivala writes that *namaste* "is an acknowledgement of the soul in one by the soul in another." The simple, heartfelt gesture of *namaste* sums up the deepest gift that yoga offers—we are all God's creatures living out God's will on earth.

Practicing yoga alongside our faith teaches us to pause and consider the idea of *namaste* as we interact with each other. This loving-kindness makes our days brighter and our relationships more rewarding.

Mind, Spirit, AND Body

Beloved, I pray that all may go well with you and that you may be in good health, just as it is well with your soul. —3 John 1:2

One aspect that sets yoga apart from other spiritual practices is its incorporation of the physical. Spirituality, at least for us in the United States, tends to be reserved for our intellects and our hearts. By incorporating the body into a spiritual practice, yoga makes it natural to incorporate spirituality into our daily, active lives. Yoga is a tool that helps us move our spiritual lives from the intangible to the tangible.

For many of us, when we first recognize a craving to develop a spiritual self, it is hard to figure out how to bring our faith and relationship to God out of church and into the "real world." With its emphasis on the body, yoga helps expand our faith from the mind and heart to body and actions.

Scripture explores this expansion of faith into life. In 1 John 3:18, we read, "Let us love, not in word or speech, but in truth and action." Showing up in church on Sundays or kneeling down to pray once a day are only the first steps to developing a full spiritual life with practices that support and strengthen us in our real-world lives. Most of us need spiritual practices that help us incorporate our faith into everything we do during the course of our day, from working on a project to talking with a friend or caring for a child.

We are always in our body. We are always breathing and moving. Practicing yoga helps us connect our physical actions to our spiritual yearnings and intentions. We learn to live our faith all the time. Yoga starts with the body—the way we carry ourselves, the way we breathe—for just this reason.

When we practice yoga, we are learning to yoke—to connect—our minds, bodies, and spirits. We are not created to be purely intellectual or purely emotional or purely physical. We can only live into our fullest selves by developing all of these aspects of ourselves.

The Yamas and Niyamas

> *Do not forsake her, and she will keep you; love her, and she will guard you. The beginning of wisdom is this: Get wisdom, and whatever else you get, get insight.*
> —Proverbs 4:6-7

This book focuses on three of yoga's eight limbs (or components): the *yamas*, the *niyamas*, and *asana*. While the Sanskrit names sound exotic, the practices themselves are quite accessible. *Asana* is the name for the yoga postures we do on our mats. The *yamas* and *niyamas* focus on principles to help guide our relationships with others and with ourselves.

The *yamas* and *niyamas* can serve as a bridge between our yoga mats and our lives. They help bring our faith out of Sunday morning worship and into every day of the week.

The Yamas

The *yamas* make up half of yoga's moral code. The Sanskrit word of *yamas* is typically translated as "moral restraints." However, the word restraint sounds, well, restrictive! Instead, think of the *yamas* as practices that help keep our actions in line with our hopes or intentions for the ways we want to live. When we allow the yamas to serve as the foundations for our actions, we find ourselves in a better place in our relationships and even with ourselves.

The five *yamas* are:
- *ahimsa* (nonviolence)
- *satya* (truthfulness)
- *asteya* (non-stealing)
- *bramacarya* (moderation)
- *aparigraha* (non-possessiveness or non-hoarding)

These principles are not unique to yoga; in fact, the *yamas* reflect the very heart of the Christian faith. In Ephesians, Paul describes how to live a life of faith. In the passage below, we have noted in brackets how Paul's words correlate with yoga's *yamas*. Our Christian faith can be strengthened through abiding by the *yamas*, these moral restraints.

> *So then, putting away falsehood, let all of us speak the truth to our neighbors, for we are members of one another* [satya]. *Be angry but do not sin; do not let the sun go down on your anger, and do not make room for the devil* [bramacarya and aparigraha]. *Thieves must give up stealing* [asteya]; *rather let them labor and work honestly with their own hands, so as to have something to share with the needy* [aparigraha]. *Let no evil talk come out of your mouths* [ahimsa], *but only what is useful for building up, as there is need, so that your words may give grace to those who hear...Put away from you all bitterness and wrath and anger and wrangling and slander, together with all malice, and be kind to one another, tender-hearted, forgiving one another* [aparigraha], *as God in Christ has forgiven you.*
> —Ephesians 5:17-32

The Niyamas
The five *niyamas* make up the second half of yoga's moral code. They are:
- *sauca* (purity)
- *santosa* (contentment)
- *tapas* (zeal)
- *svadhyaya* (self-study)
- *isvara-pranidhana* (devotion to God)

The Sanskrit word *niyamas* is traditionally defined as "observances." Practicing the *niyamas* supports the changes that we've made in our lives by the *yamas*. The *niyamas* provide an instruction manual of sorts. They essentially describe how to put into action the beliefs expressed in the *yamas*. The *niyamas* take us from the conceptual to the actual. The *niyamas* describe how to bring our spirituality into our real-world lives.

The *niyamas* are practices that have been found, over thousands of years, to support the individual who has chosen a spiritual path. Sharath Jois, in his book *Astanga Yoga Anusthana*, defines the *niyamas* as commitments we make to ourselves. That's worth repeating and considering. They are commitments we make to ourselves—they are not imposed on us or required of us. The *niyamas* are yoga's invitation to choose a different path in life. They are yoga's invitation to draw closer to God every single day.

As you work through this guide, it will become clear that the *yamas* and *niyamas* are braided together and support one another. For example, a practice of *sauca* (purity or cleanliness) requires an element of *satya* (truthfulness) and *tapas* (passion or zeal). In order to recognize that you've made a mess of something (whether tangible or intangible), you must be clear-eyed and honest with yourself. You also must apply yourself with determination and zeal to the work of cleaning up after yourself.

A Practice of Transformation

> *This is what I have seen to be good: it is fitting to eat and drink and find enjoyment in all the toil with which one toils under the sun the few days of the life God gives us; for this is our lot.* —Ecclesiastes 5:18

Yoga has a curious, circular nature. Each limb is like a spoke on a wheel. Each spoke serves to make the whole practice stronger. We can work on each limb within our practices of any of the other limbs. Working with our bodies on our mats in *asana* provides a wonderful laboratory to experiment and practice with the moral teachings of yoga before applying them in real life. After all of this practice, putting these moral tenets to use in our daily life becomes second nature.

Our physical practice helps to weave these moral tenets into the very cloth of who we are. We will still face challenges and have obligations and chores, good days and bad. The adoption of a spiritual practice like yoga isn't a lucky coin or panacea. Rather, spiritual practices transform our approach to life. An old Zen saying reinforces this point: "Before enlightenment, I chopped wood and carried water. After enlightenment, I chopped wood and carried water."

We can't control what life brings our way. We can only control our response to the chances and changes of life. A spiritual disciple of prayer, reflection, and practice can help us find enjoyment even in toil and tribulation and to discover deeper meaning in all we do.

Day 1
Ahimsa/Nonviolence

Pray

Eternal God, in whose perfect kingdom no sword is drawn but the sword of righteousness, no strength known but the strength of love: So mightily spread abroad your Spirit, that all peoples may be gathered under the banner of the Prince of Peace, as children of one Father; to whom be dominion and glory, now and forever. Amen. —The Book of Common Prayer

Reflect

The concept of *ahimsa* asks us to embrace nonviolence at the levels of speech, thought, and action. It means not causing harm to other living beings. Violence is a loaded word, isn't it? It makes us think of guns, beatings, and warfare. It is important that we stretch beyond this understanding of what it means to commit acts of violence.

Violence can take on many forms. Some forms of violence are obvious. Others are less obvious. For instance, unkind words can hurt feelings, destroy self-esteem, undermine confidence, and radically change the direction of an individual's life or the life of a relationship.

Some forms of violence are even sneakier. Thoughts fall squarely into this category. We all maintain an inner dialogue as we evaluate and judge our actions over the course of the day. It's not uncommon for people to be totally unconscious of this audio loop in our heads. And sometimes, we are not kind to ourselves. Chances are, our inner voice may be among the cruelest voices we will ever hear. We can wreak violence on ourselves, and this kind of self-violence is deeply damaging. This is a habit or pattern that we need to notice. And, by noticing it, we can begin to change it.

Today as you practice, notice how you treat your body and the words you are saying about yourself while on your mat. Are you pushing yourself too hard in a way that might lead to injury? Are you being overly critical of your perceived lack of progress to obtain a goal you had hoped you would reach by now? Today's invitation is to end this violence—whether it be on your mat or in the world—by ending it first in yourself.

Practice

Turn to page 50 and move through the sun salutation and other poses. As you practice, consider the principle of *ahimsa*. When we are nonviolent, others around us will cease to be hostile. That's a big promise, isn't it? Can we really change the world by changing our own behavior? Jesus thought so. Gandhi thought so, too. So did Martin Luther King Jr., Mother Teresa, Rosa Parks, and Nelson Mandela, to name just a few.

When we go through life with an awareness of the ways our words, thoughts, and deeds could potentially harm others or ourselves, the feelings of love and connectedness that arise are astounding. As we begin to practice, we should be aware of the ripple effect of each thought, word, and deed. Practicing *ahimsa* helps us reject the illusion of separateness and accept the reality that we are all deeply connected to one another. As we practice *ahimsa*, we move ever closer to the understanding that we are enacting love when we practice nonviolence. This love is the tie that binds us all together.

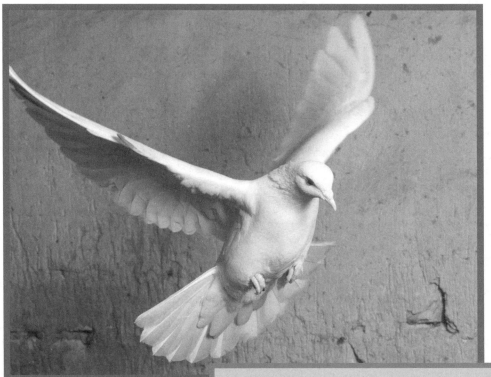

Ahimsapratisthayam tat sannidhau vairatyagah YS2:35
When we live nonviolently, those around us cease to be violent.

Day 2
Ahimsa/Nonviolence

Pray

Most holy God, the source of all good desires, all right judgments, and all just works: Give to us, your servants, that peace which the world cannot give, so that our minds may be fixed on the doing of your will, and that we, being delivered from the fear of all enemies, may live in peace and quietness; through the mercies of Christ Jesus our Savior. Amen.
—*The Book of Common Prayer*

Reflect

Peacefulness or nonviolence encompasses much of Jesus' message to his followers. Nonviolence is at the foundation of Jesus' greatest commandment, "Love one another. Just as I have loved you, you also should love one another." In other words, living responsible, moral lives—living as good citizens—requires that we do not hurt one another.

Jesus did not simply talk about peace—he lived it. So often, when Jesus was approached by people who wanted him to be a militaristic messiah, one who came to liberate his people with a mighty sword, he gave them an answer of an all-encompassing love rather than a call to violence. He pointed to God's desire to save and free all people through him rather than a desire for gold or riches or power that would come at the price of leaving others suffering or in want.

For Jesus, the only reign he would usher in was one of peace, free from the violence we so readily inflict on one another. By commanding us to love one another, Jesus is telling us that we are to take up his call to nonviolence and to spread peace and love in his name.

Practice

One of the ways we can begin to spread this kind of love is through prayer and peaceful actions such as yoga. As you move through the poses on pages 50-81, spend some time thinking about the peace and the love that you could spread in all ways. For example, on the mat, you might practice this intention by approaching a posture you hate with gratitude for the way your body will change through it. Spend a few extra moments in this posture, breathing love into the frustration you have with it.

Or as you find yourself having violent thoughts, actions, or words off the mat, remember that if your first lens is one of love, you will be less inclined to choose violence as a responsive action. Take the same calming breaths before reacting to invite love and peace into your heart at that moment.

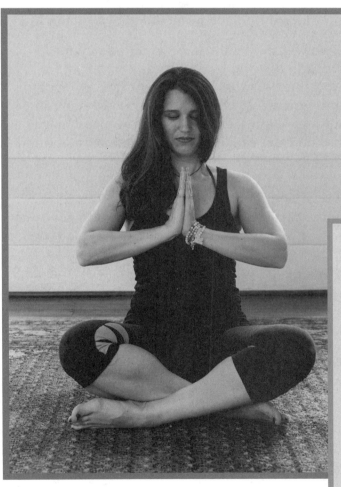

A Few Deep Breaths

The opening breaths of your practice are very important and very powerful. Close your eyes. Tune out all outside distractions. (We know. This feels weird.) Just breathe. Try not to change your breathing. Simply observe it. Notice if you are inhaling or exhaling. What does each breath feel like? Can you feel the cool air as your breath flows in? Can you feel the warmth of your breath as you exhale? Have you noticed that your mind has slowed down and your emotions have smoothed out, all as a result of simply focusing on your breath? This is just a taste of the power of mindful breathing.

Day 3
Ahimsa/Nonviolence

Pray

O God, you manifest in your servants the signs of your presence: Send forth upon us the Spirit of love, that in companionship with one another your abounding grace may increase among us; through Jesus Christ our Lord. Amen. —*The Book of Common Prayer*

Reflect

As we mentioned in the introduction, we will spend three days on each yoga principle. One day we will look at it through a yogic lens, one day through a Christian lens, and the third day through the personal lens of experience. Today is the first of those introspective days, and you are invited to spend time reflecting on what the Holy Spirit is doing in your life. We have provided a prompt for contemplation and invite you to journal on how your soul and practice have been opened up by each principle.

Reflect upon these two famous quotations, one from Jesus as he delivered the Sermon on the Mount and the other from Martin Luther King Jr., whose embrace of nonviolent protest inspired a nation.

Blessed are the peacemakers, for they will be called children of God.—Matthew 5:9

God, help us as individuals and as a world to hear it now before it is too late: "Seek ye first the Kingdom of God and God's justice and all these other things shall be added unto you."—Martin Luther King Jr.

How could you bring more *ahimsa* into your practice? How could you bring more of it into the world?

Practice

On this final day centered on *ahimsa*, consider practices that you can use to focus on Christ's commandment to love, in your life on and off the mat. Here are three suggestions:

- Today, when you notice yourself having harsh thoughts about something you've said or done, spend a moment editing these thoughts into a kinder version.
- During your practice, every time you inhale deeply, allow that breath to fill you with a healing feeling. Allow each exhale to serve as a release of any negativity you find within your heart or mind.
- Explore your own experiences with *ahimsa* in your journal.

You may have other practices that you would like to exercise as you embrace the principle of *ahimsa*/nonviolence. However you strive to live out this principle, invite Jesus to be with you in this endeavor to live spiritually.

_____

_____

_____

_____

_____

_____

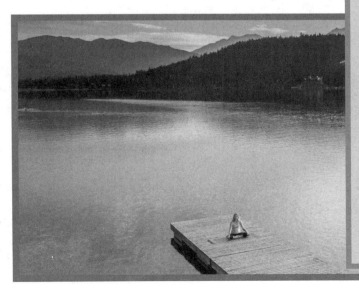

Holding Still Is Hard to Do

It is a bit of a paradox that all the movement of yoga is designed to teach us to hold still, inside and out. If you feel jumpy as you begin, you're not alone. Most of us struggle mightily to hold still, especially when we have been told to hold still! Trust us here. Your practice will take care of your need to fidget. When you reach *savasana* or resting pose at the end of your practice and enter into meditation, you will be surprised at how willing your body is to truly, deeply rest. Your still body will serve as a roadmap for your mind as it journeys toward its own stillness.

Day 4
Satya/Truthfulness

Pray

Almighty and everlasting God, mercifully increase in us your gifts of holy discipline, in almsgiving, prayer, and practice; that our lives may be directed to the fulfilling of your most gracious will; through Jesus Christ our Lord, who lives and reigns with you and the Holy Spirit, one God, for ever and ever. Amen.
—Lesser Feasts and Fasts

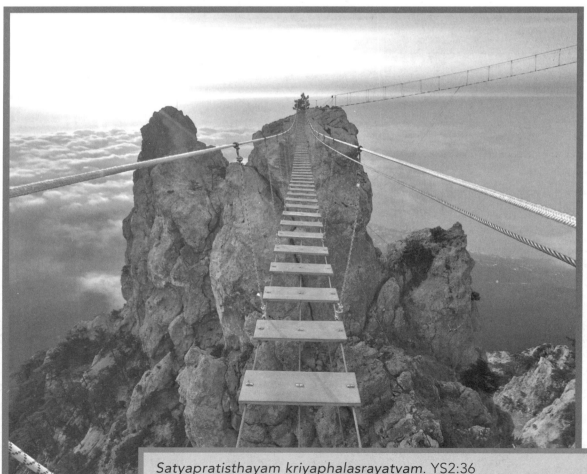

Satyapratisthayam kriyaphalasrayatvam. YS2:36
When we are truthful, whatever action we take will be successful.

Reflect

Satya means being truthful. It is natural for us to immediately think of words when we are discussing truthfulness and honesty. But *satya* goes further than that, asking us to be truthful in our thoughts and actions as well.

To begin with the word aspect of *satya*, telling the truth doesn't mean simply avoiding bald-faced lies but also refraining from embellishments or minimizations, omissions, and rationalizations. Untruthfulness can take many different forms and have many different motivations. Even a little exaggeration can be used to gain power over someone else. A little white lie told with good intention can end up hurting just as much as a whopper. While definitely not easy, it is kinder to be honest. Today, pay close attention to your words and actions. You may be surprised by how many times in a given day you resort to (or are tempted to offer) a falsehood of some kind.

Satya is also about being truthful to ourselves in words, actions, and thoughts. Perhaps you think you can't sit in a certain yoga posture because of "tight runner's legs," but in all honesty, your reluctance to try is based in fear and not truth. Or perhaps you turn down an opportunity to work on a special project, telling yourself that you're not ready or that you don't have the skills. Be honest with yourself: Is truth or fear guiding your decision?

Satya highlights our limiting beliefs about ourselves so that we are aware of them and can question or challenge them. In the end, practicing *satya* can lead us to a broader and deeper life experience. Practicing *satya* can improve our relationships with others and ourselves. It can inspire us to stretch ourselves or give us the courage to face a challenge. Ultimately *satya* is a practice that will deepen and strengthen our spiritual lives as we begin to see and know ourselves clearly as God sees and knows us.

Practice

In your practice today, seek *satya* in each posture you hold. Are you holding each one for the full measure of the breath? Are you falling into complacency or old habits and expectations when you might be able to go further in some places? Or would going further than you can safely stretch be a dangerous lie that could cause you to get hurt? Being honest with yourself on the mat is a safe yet powerful way to begin practicing truthfulness in all parts of life.

Day 5
Satya/Truthfulness

Pray

Almighty God, to you all hearts are open, all desires known, and from you no secrets are hid: Cleanse the thoughts of our hearts by the inspiration of your Holy Spirit that we may perfectly love you, and worthily magnify your holy Name; through Christ our Lord. Amen. —The Book of Common Prayer

Reflect

In John 14:6-7, Jesus tells his followers: "I am the way, and the truth, and the life. No one comes to the Father except through me. If you know me, you will know my Father also." In other words, Jesus is telling us the importance of believing in his teachings and in the truth of his love.

The *satya*—the truth—that Jesus describes sets us free because it means that we will not be separated from Jesus, even by death. We know this truth because Jesus came to dwell with us so we could know him fully. To know Jesus is to know the love of God face-to-face. It is the truth that is bolder than any other truth because it speaks of life for all people.

When it comes to the truth, Jesus was firm in his understanding that "the truth will make you free" (John 8:32). This *satya* is the ultimate truth, not just a simplistic or naive truth. It is not a "the truth is I love pizza" kind of truth. That might be completely the case, but a love of pizza will never set you free in a grand way. No, Jesus is describing an all-encompassing and life-changing truth that points us to God's love for us.

Sometimes we think of humility and truth-telling as a somber endeavor, perhaps one that requires a great deal of time in repentance mode. Yet, when we spend time dwelling in God's *satya*, it is impossible not to be thrilled with the liberating power of God's desire to be with us. Telling the truth means living and breathing good news!

Practice

In your practice today, pay attention to postures that express your thankfulness for God's *satya*. Perhaps you will express this gratitude in chest opener postures (such as bridge pose found on pages 76-77) that show an open heart for God. Or maybe you will spend more time in a meditation pose (such as ones on pages 80-81) to dwell on the freedom-giving truth you know in Jesus. Let your body sing out an Alleluia as you give thanks for God's unfailing *satya*.

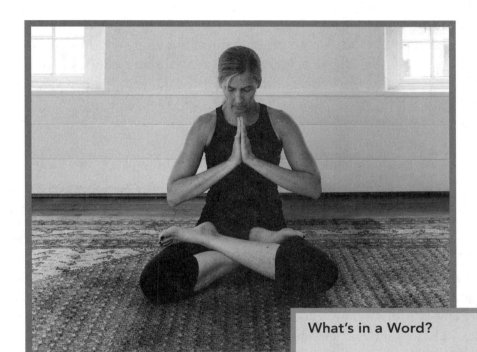

What's in a Word?

As you explore the world of yoga, there are a few words you will often hear. *Om* is said to be the sound of the energetic vibration of the universe that we could hear if everything else were silent. *Shanti* means peace. *Namaste* is a greeting that means the light and good in me recognizes and bows to the light and good in you.

Day 6
Satya/Truthfulness

Pray

Bless us, O God, in this holy time, in which our hearts seek your help and healing; and so purify us by your discipline that we may grow in grace, in truth, and in the knowledge of our Lord and Savior Jesus Christ; who lives and reigns with you and the Holy Spirit, one God, forever and ever. Amen.
—Lesser Feasts and Fasts

Reflect

On this, the final day centered on *satya*, our hope is that you will explore truthfulness more deeply. How have you begun to see your life or your practice changing to match your intentions? How has God begun to work in all aspects of your life?

Let yourself be truthful with God as well as yourself. Ironically, we tend to hide our true self from God who knows everything about us and that means we cannot be fully present with God. Let us sit assured in the belief that God does not love us because we are good—God loves us because God is good and we do not need to hide ourselves with obfuscation or lies.

At the same time, we must balance our truth telling with an awareness of how our words and actions may affect others. Some truths are better left unsaid. For example, while we may think a friend's haircut is atrocious, offering an honest assessment would be hurtful. In some situations, we may need to speak a truth that will cause pain—with the hope that healing and wholeness will follow. The *yamas* of *satya* (truthfulness) should work hand in hand with the *yamas* of *ahimsa* (nonviolence). Yoga teaches us that balance is key, in both our physical and spiritual practices. We must learn to honor all of the *yamas*—and keep quiet about that haircut.

Practice

- The 12-step recovery program is a familiar concept for many. As we consider living the truthful life, spending time with these steps may help us to do so. For today's meditation, we can consider Steps 4, 8, and 9. Step 4 encourages participants to make a fearless moral inventory. We can consider the lies we've told in the last week and truly examine those incidents. Merging Steps 8 and 9, we can then make a list of people hurt by those lies and make amends with them (or ourselves), as we are able.
- Ask your partner, a family member, or a close friend to tell you a truth that he or she has never shared with you. Then do the same in return.
- Explore your own experiences with *satya* in your journal.
- No matter how you engage the practice of *satya*, ask Jesus to be with you every breath you take. As you move through the poses, pray for Jesus to be with you during each inhale of breath. Thank Jesus for his presence each time you exhale.

Demystifying Sanskrit

By now, you have probably noticed that yoga is associated with another language—and the words in that other language are really long! The language used in the traditional names of yoga postures and in the original text of the *sutras* is Sanskrit. It is from India. These Sanskrit words are compound words, which is why they look so long. When you learn a few of the words, Sanskrit begins to seem a little less intimidating. Here are a few that you've seen in our series of postures: *asana*=seat or posture; *tri*=three; *hasta*=holding on to; *kona*=angle; *utthita*=extended; *sirsa*=head; *sava*=corpse; *surya*=sun; *namaskar*=greeting or salutation. So, for instance when you see the word *savasana*, it means "corpse posture."

Pray

Almighty God, the fountain of all wisdom, you know our necessities before we ask and our ignorance in asking: Have compassion on our weakness, and mercifully give us those things which for our unworthiness we dare not, and for our blindness we cannot ask; through the worthiness of your Son Jesus Christ our Lord, who lives and reigns with you and the Holy Spirit, one God, now and for ever. Amen.
—The Book of Common Prayer

Reflect

Let's start with the obvious: We shouldn't take things that belong to someone else. This is a lesson we were taught early in life. But that doesn't mean this *yama* is always easy to follow. Most of us don't have a problem with outright theft. We don't shoplift or cash fraudulent checks or break into homes.

But there are plenty of ways that we steal. We make the choice to keep the $10 in change a harried cashier at the store gives us instead of a single dollar. Windfall! We habitually overstay our allotted session with a therapist. We cheat ("just a little") on our taxes. We "forget" to return our sister's awesome sweater that she left in our apartment the last time she visited.

It is also possible to steal things we can't hold or touch. We take credit for work done by someone else or we plagiarize, presenting someone else's thoughts and words as our own. Stealing can occur in many different ways.

We need to consider our motivations to steal. In some cases, it's simply desire. We see something, we want it, and we take it. In many situations, stealing is motivated by a belief that there is not enough in the world to go around. We believe that if we don't grab it (money, objects, undue credit), we'll be left without. This assumption of scarcity makes it easy for us to rationalize stealing.

When we operate from a place of scarcity, we focus on what we do not have rather than being mindful of and thankful for what we do have. A fundamental shift in outlook from scarcity to abundance can be life-altering. By focusing on all we have in life, our attitudes shift to joy, gratitude, and contentment. A shift in outlook takes practice, dedication, and effort.

How do we make this shift? We trust. We practice gratitude. We have faith. In fact, faith may be the most important key in making this shift in perspective. We develop a deep confidence that our needs will be met. According to the prophets of the Old Testament, the stories and parables of Jesus, and the teachings of ancient yogis, there is no treasure greater than the peace of mind and ultimate joy that we attain through spending dedicated time meditating on and with God.

Practice

As you practice today, notice where you are stealing from yourself. On days when you feel sluggish, take a closer look. Are you truly worn out or are you being lazy? By embracing a grateful heart, you can tap into stores of energy that can keep you going and the desire to stop will start to melt away. Look for areas of theft in your life and practice *asteya* instead.

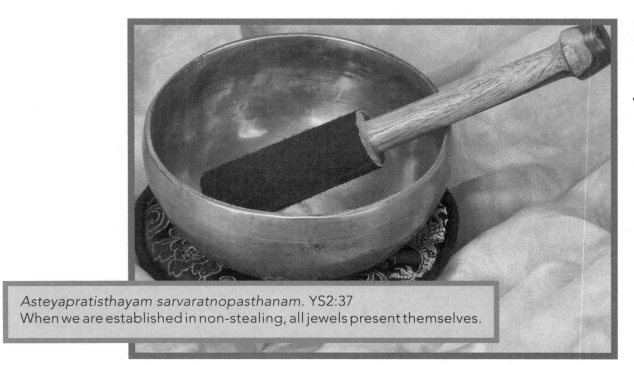

Asteyapratisthayam sarvaratnopasthanam. YS2:37
When we are established in non-stealing, all jewels present themselves.

Day 8
Asteya/Non-Stealing

Pray

Lord Christ, our eternal Redeemer, grant us such fellowship in your sufferings, that, filled with your Holy Spirit, we may subdue the flesh to the spirit, and the spirit to you, and at the last attain to the glory of your resurrection; who lives and reigns with the Father and the Holy Spirit, one God, for ever and ever. Amen.
—Lesser Feasts and Fasts

Reflect

As we continue to explore *asteya* or non-stealing, we must keep in mind the root of theft is the worry of not enough. This worry can stand in the way of our relationship with God and, ironically, starts stealing our peace.

God wants us to know peace that extends beyond our worry on what we do not have. In one of the most beloved passages of scripture, Psalm 23, we hear these words: "The LORD is my shepherd; I shall not be in want." Here, God is loving and protecting us, promising to meet our deepest needs. Yes, we may experience valleys and shadows, situations that are hard and dark, but our Lord God abides with us always. When we truly believe this, we come to understand that there is enough love for everyone. We do not have to jealously search for it in a neighbor's pasture. We have all we need.

In the Gospel of Matthew, Jesus urges us to lay our worries aside. Jesus preaches: "Do not worry, saying 'What will we eat?' or 'What will we drink?' or 'What will we wear?'...Strive first for the kingdom of God and his righteousness, and all these things will be given to you as well" (6:31-33).

Jesus is describing a peace that comes when we let go of the worry that we will not have enough. When we worry we don't have enough, we look to get more at any cost, even stealing. When we steal, we add a new worry, the worry of being caught. Jesus tells us that God will provide for our every need. Trust in that truth can be liberating and life-giving.

Practice

When we seek to practice this trust, we can again gain insight from our practice and our prayers. When we trust the practice to change us over time, we have a peace that we will arrive where we should when we should. However, when we perceive a lack (like inflexibility or weakness), we can become worried and anxious and may even lose our motivation.

In your practice today, ask God to calm your hearts and dwell in the peace that comes with trusting God.

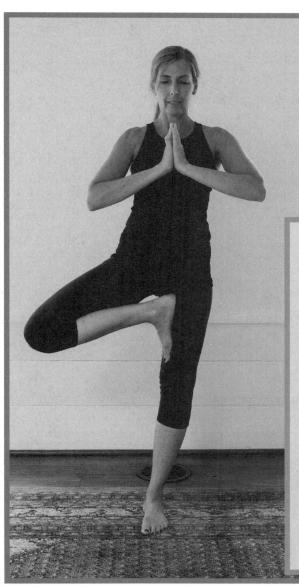

Practicing with Fear

We all feel fear. It is sometimes a surprise to the new yoga student how often fear crops up in a yoga practice. Yoga teaches us there are two types of fear: fear that keeps us safe and fear that holds us back or keeps us stuck. As your practice grows and develops, you will face fear. You will be able to use the deepening awareness that your practice is creating to discern whether the fear you are feeling is keeping you safe or holding you back. If it is the first type, we encourage you to honor that fear and hold off on the posture. If it is the second type however, we invite you to take a deep breath and try. You may have to do this several (or a hundred!) times. It is your willingness to try that will cause your fear to shrink and even disappear.

Day 9
Asteya/Non-Stealing

Pray

O God, by your Word you marvelously carry out the work of reconciliation: Grant that in our prayerful journey we may be devoted to you with all our hearts, and united with one another in prayer and holy love; through Jesus Christ our Lord, who lives and reigns with you and the Holy Spirit, one God, for ever and ever. Amen. —Lesser Feasts and Fasts, amended

Reflect

As mentioned earlier, we may not notice the prevalence of stealing in our behavior until we stop and consider the smaller thefts that happen in our lives. How has your understanding of this *yama* changed over the last few days? How is it important to you? What do you feel is its intention?

_____

_____

_____

_____

_____

_____

_____

_____

_____

Practice

Today, we wrap up our consideration of *asteya* or non-stealing. It is especially important that we take time to truly look at our life to find moments of theft that might otherwise go without notice. By reflecting on *asteya*, we not only free ourselves from the sin of stealing but also build trust in our generous God who wishes to provide for us. Here are a few suggestions to help explore your practice (or lack thereof) of *asteya*:

- Write down how you spend your time each day. Are there gaps of time that are being used for pleasure rather than contracted work? These might be places that need to be reevaluated. Ask yourself why you might be stealing time from others.
- Look at your prayer life. What kind of concerns are you bringing to God? If you lift your worries in prayer, God will hear them and help you not carry them with you, serving as a temptation to steal.
- Practice the ancient monastic practice of the beggar's bowl. It was an exercise in relying totally on God. When the monks would leave the monastery every day, they would carry with them only a small bowl and no food, trusting that God would provide them with the sustenance they would need. Try this for a day to help shine light on all that you have to be grateful for.
- Explore your experiences with *asteya* in your journal.

When to Practice

Traditionally yoga is practiced as you begin your day, after your morning ablutions (washing up) and before your morning meal. That said, your practice must fit into the rhythms of your life in order to be sustainable. If your early morning hours are full to the brim, you may need to look for another time. The lunch hour can be a great time to practice, fortifying you to better weather a mid-afternoon energy slump. Evenings can be very restorative times to practice, helping you to release any stresses, tensions, and worries of your day before you settle in for your rest. If you try a time of day and it does not "stick," try another. You'll find the right time for you to practice.

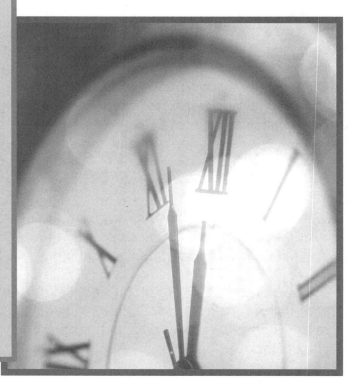

Day 10
Bramacarya/Temperance

Pray

O God, whose blessed Son became poor that we through his poverty might be rich: Deliver us from an inordinate love of this world, that we, inspired by the devotion of your servant, may serve you with singleness of heart, and attain to the riches of the age to come; through Jesus Christ our Lord, who lives and reigns with you, in the unity of the Holy Spirit, one God, now and for ever. Amen. —The Book of Common Prayer

Reflect

Bramacarya is about finding balance. We seek balance and moderation in a world that is wildly out of balance. Every day, we are bombarded by the message that we are "in need" by commercials touting the latest tools or toys or luxuries that will make our lives easier, better, happier. We are told over and over again that "stuff" can make us happy.

Desire and imbalance can affect almost every aspect of our lives. Some of us struggle with too much work; others with too much play. Some of us have unhealthy relationships with food, causing us to lose touch with our bodies' messages of hunger and to eat (or not eat) as an emotional refuge. Some of us can be overly fixated on exercise, craving "more, more, more!" of the endorphin buzz we get from a long run. Others of us can get obsessive over a hobby (gardening, reading, even yoga!) to the point that it consumes more than its fair share of our time. In all of these cases, immoderation takes our energy away from other areas in our lives. It causes imbalance.

A conscious act of will is required to tune out these messages. The constant, chattering commercial of more draws our attention away from all that we have. When we allow that chant of "more" to run amok, we risk losing the joy we have in our lives.

When we embark on a spiritual practice of *bramacarya*, we are being countercultural. We are choosing to resist a culture of overindulgence and to embrace a simpler life. We may come to realize that our happiest existence might be achieved through balance and moderation.

Yoga philosophy teaches that desire is at the root of almost all discontent. It's easy to convince ourselves if we could just have "that," then we would be happy. But the reality is nothing outside of ourselves can make us happy. Peace and joy are already ours. We simply have to connect with the peace and joy deep within ourselves. Like *asteya, bramacarya* shifts our viewpoint from one of need to one of abundance. It relies on the belief that God will meet all our needs—and not necessarily all our wants. The key is to develop the ability to tell the difference!

Practice

Grateful moderation can certainly be practiced on our mats. So often we come to our practice thinking that we must do more and more. We might find ourselves saying, "If I could just twist further!" or "If I could only bend forward more!" as expressions of our discontentment with our current state. This discontentment can lead to injury and a painful feeling of lack. *Bramacarya* invites us to let go of those desires and preconceived notions so that we might fully live in the moment and be grateful for the gifts we have received. Today as you practice, celebrate each posture as it is today—perfectly enough to restore your body, mind, and spirit.

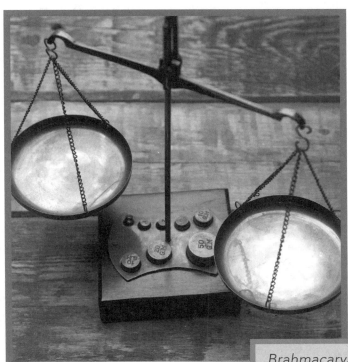

Brahmacaryapratishayam viryalabhah. YS2:38
When we practice moderation, we will have vigor, valor, and energy.

Day 11
Bramacarya/Temperance

Pray

> O God, you willed to redeem us from all iniquity by
> your Son: Deliver us when we are tempted to regard
> sin without abhorrence, and let the virtue of his passion
> come between us and our mortal enemies; through
> Jesus Christ our Lord, who lives and reigns with you
> and the Holy Spirit, one God, for ever and ever. Amen.
> —Lesser Feasts and Fasts

Reflect

As we continue our exploration of *bramacarya*, let us reflect on the story of Jesus
being tempted by Satan in the desert. Satan tempts Jesus with invitations to more—
more food, more power, more control over the will of God. These are all within Jesus'
grasp, if he will just turn to Satan. But Jesus answers these temptations by saying:
"One does not live by bread alone, but every word that comes from the mouth of
God" (Matthew 4:4). In other words, Jesus is clear that nothing is as delicious or
powerful or wonderful as God's love. And we already have God's love. We need not
chase our desires, as they will only lead us away from the knowledge of that love.

We may not believe we are strong enough to resist those things that tempt us the
most. The problem with this thinking is that it makes it seem like we simply need
more willpower to rise above these temptations. The truth is that willpower is finite in
all of us. Even the strongest monk will tell you that dealing with temptation is more
about avoiding than resisting it. At the end of his encounter with Satan, Jesus tells
him to leave—sending Satan and his temptations far away. Jesus was practicing a
type of *bramacarya* by removing the tempter's power.

Practice

As you seek to apply this Christ-like *bramacarya* in your life, start your practice
today admitting to and listing the things that tempt you. Do you desire power,
things, or a person's love? Once you have listed them, hand them over to God
(perhaps using the prayer above). Pray to replace the desire for more through the
lens of this intention, then ask yourself: Was the practice any different having rid
yourself of imbalance and immoderation?

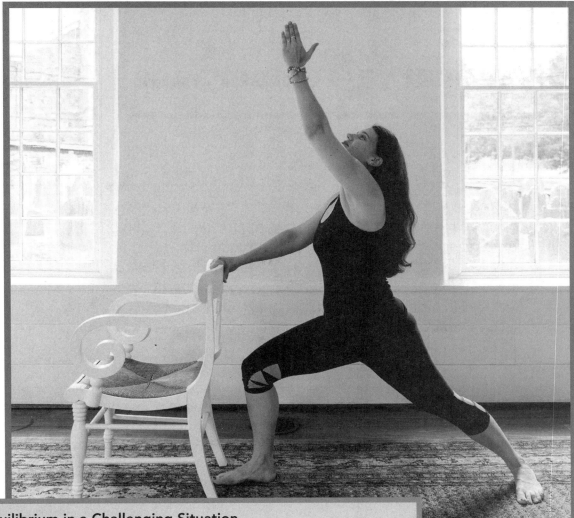

Equilibrium in a Challenging Situation

The challenges we face on our yoga mats—a lunge that is hard to sustain or a balance that is a struggle to maintain—are metaphors for the challenges that life brings our way. On our mats, we learn to take one breath at a time. We learn to relax our clenched jaw or toes. We learn to celebrate what we can do. We learn to fall down (or step out early) gracefully. And we learn to try again (and again and again). These excellent life skills will carry us through challenging situations with poise and equanimity.

Day 12
Bramacarya/Temperance

Pray

> *O merciful Creator, your hand is open wide to satisfy the needs of every living creature: Make us always thankful for your loving providence; and grant that we, remembering the account that we must one day give, may be faithful stewards of your good gifts; through Jesus Christ our Lord, who with you and the Holy Spirit lives and reigns, one God, for ever and ever.* Amen.
> —The Book of Common Prayer

Reflect

In your refection time today, begin to identify the ways you have already experienced *bramacarya* on this journey. Remember your experiences in practice are more than your physical actions. Consider your thoughts, your inner "narrator," and your reactions to the exercise. Where are you feeling the need to move into moderation or where has it already started to happen?

Practice

As we conclude our exploration of *bramacarya*, let us again turn to ways we can practice this all-important *yama* on and off our mat. Remember that the intention is about letting go of desire and embracing the peace that comes from dependence on a good and loving God. Consider these suggestions for letting go of different kinds of desires:

- As you listen to the radio or watch TV, pay attention to your reactions to advertisements. Count how many ads you are exposed to during a 15-minute period, including hidden ads such as product placements in a show. Notice feelings of false desire that rise up in you as a result of these ads. Try working with your breath during each ad, inhaling peace and contentment, exhaling desire.
- When the occasion arises, go along with what your partner or friend wants. Let her pick the restaurant or movie. Or, if you always rely on him to lead, you pick. Relinquish the habit of having to be in charge or the habit of giving in.
- Explore your own experiences with *bramacarya* in your journal.

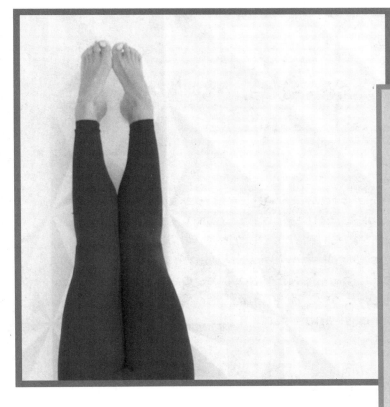

Therapeutic Benefits of Yoga

Yoga *asanas* (postures) have many therapeutic benefits beyond opening tight muscles. Twists release tight muscles in the back as well as tension and stress from a busy day or rough time of life. Forward folds massage the abdominal organs, which yields better digestive health. Postures that create more range of motion in the hips can strengthen the low back and reduce knee pain. Inversions increase cardiovascular health and flood the brain with fresh, oxygenated, nutrient-rich blood for better mental health.

Day 13
Aparigraha/Non-Possessiveness

Pray

> Almighty and most merciful God, drive from us all weakness of body, mind, and spirit; that, being restored to wholeness, we may with free hearts become what you intend us to be and accomplish what you want us to do; through Jesus Christ our Lord, who lives and reigns with you and the Holy Spirit, one God, for ever and ever. Amen. —Lesser Feast and Fasts

Reflect

Aparigraha is often translated as "non-possessiveness" or even "non-hoarding." Non-possessiveness teaches us to give generously of all we are and all we have. Non-possessiveness teaches us to put our resources to work now. Living into *aparigraha* requires a level of faith that our needs will be met on a future "rainy day."

In Christian scripture we are encouraged to make caring for the needy our priority. We are taught that God loves a cheerful giver.

> The one who sows sparingly will also reap sparingly, and the one who sows bountifully will also reap bountifully. Each of you must give as you have made up your mind, not reluctantly or under compulsion, for God loves a cheerful giver. And God is able to provide you with every blessing in abundance, so that by always having enough of everything, you may share abundantly in every good work. —2 Corinthians 9:6-8

We are taught that all that we have and all that we are is a gift from God and that God intends us to "re-gift" these treasures!

When we come to our mats, greed often awaits us there. We desire to go further in our postures. We desire to be able to have the grace and flow that we perceive in our neighbor's practice. We want to control our bodies and our minds to achieve the heights we want. Yet, this kind of greed forces us to forget the journey we have already been blessed with in our bodies, the intention of the present moment, or to revel in the promise of where our practice will go. Today, allow yourself to be satisfied with the gifts of each posture as they come—and let go of the desire for more.

Aparigraha is also about letting go and can be practiced at a very tangible, mundane level. For example, you are practicing *aparigraha* when you purge old clothes from your closet or books from your shelf. When the work is done, when you've parted ways with belongings you no longer want or need, you might find yourself feeling elated. Letting go feels good.

Finally, *aparigraha* frees us to take a look at where we're grasping onto ideas and beliefs that should be released. It allows us to be interested in who we are today. The only thing we can be certain of is that we are different today than we were yesterday—and will be tomorrow. Until we let go of our old ideas, we will not be able to receive the gifts of *aparigraha*.

Practice

On our yoga mats, we find one of the greatest gifts that *aparigraha* offers is "beginner's mind." Operate today from a beginner's mind. Approach each *asana* (yoga posture) with curiosity and interest. This perspective allows us to release our assumptions about what we can or can't do. We come to our mats fresh. We find out in the moment what feels right for our bodies. Quite frequently, our bodies will surprise us, and our practices will seem as fresh and exciting as they were the first day we wandered onto our mats.

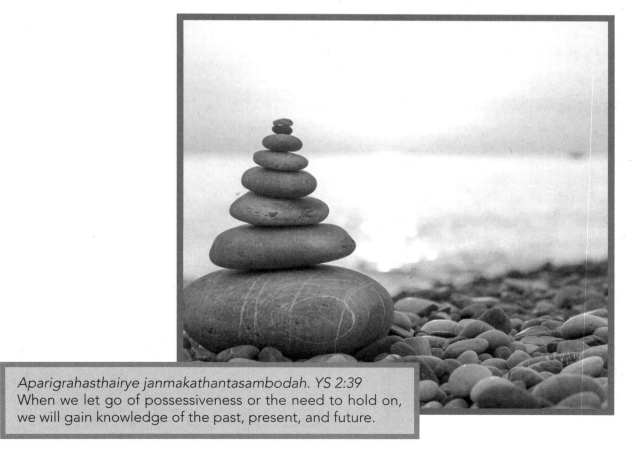

Aparigrahasthairye janmakathantasambodah. YS 2:39
When we let go of possessiveness or the need to hold on, we will gain knowledge of the past, present, and future.

Day 14
Aparigraha/Non-Possessiveness

Pray

Grant, O Lord, that as your Son Jesus Christ prayed for his enemies on the cross, so we may have grace to forgive those who wrongfully or scornfully use us, that we ourselves may be able to receive your forgiveness; through Jesus Christ our Lord, who lives and reigns with you and the Holy Spirit, one God, forever and ever. Amen. —Lesser Feasts and Fasts

Reflect

We are all guilty of spiritual hoarding—that is, withholding forgiveness. In the Gospel of Matthew, Peter asks Jesus about forgiveness: "'Lord, if another member of the church sins against me, how often should I forgive? As many as seven times?' Jesus said to him, 'Not seven times, but, I tell you, seventy-seven times'" (18:21-22). In Jesus' view, forgiveness—relinquishing a wrong committed against you or one you committed yourself—is the key to living fully.

Clearly, forgiveness is of the utmost importance to Jesus, and he wants us to know that it is not enough to partially forgive. We must be willing to purge all the anger and frustration that burrows into our hearts when we lust after vengeance or our sense of justice. Jesus knows the truth about such spiritual hoarding—the longer we hold onto it, the more destruction it wreaks upon us. We must practice *aparigraha* and let go.

Sometimes, the pain of non-forgiving is so deep that we may not even know it is there. Yet its impact is felt in numerous ways. We may not trust easily. We may lash out without reason. We may not be able to form deep relationships. All of these reactions may be symptoms of a deep hurt that has yet to be let go.

When we are finally able to let go and forgive, we find the life that God imagines for us, one that is free from the pain of being bound up in old wounds. We feel the freedom that comes with letting go.

Practice

Today, when you are in upward facing dog or bridge pose, which opens the heart, say the prayer for this day. Spend some time feeling what rises up within you and let yourself be physically vulnerable. Don't be surprised if anger or fear or even tears spring forth. Allow your emotions to happen, notice them, and pray for the guidance to let go of what is causing them.

Setting Intention

Setting an intention before you start to move and breathe can transform your practice from a physical one to a spiritual one. Our *asana* practice is a moving prayer that draws us into an intimate time with God. As our practices have evolved over the years, we have settled into the habit of starting our practices with a prayer. There is no right or wrong way to do this. Your opening prayer can be different each time you practice; for instance, you can use the prayer we have offered in this book for each of the thirty days. Or you might settle on a prayer that feels perfect for you to use every day. It could be part of a prayer you love, part of the liturgy in your worship service, or part of a poem that opens your heart. There are as many ways to set intentions as there are people who practice yoga. Take time to find yours. It is well worth it.

Daily Practice

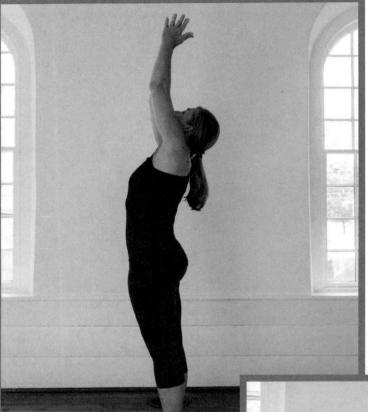

Surya Namaskar A Sun Salutations

The sun salutations are a series of movements designed to set the rhythm of your practice, to draw your mind inward, and to warm up your muscles. We recommend that you begin your daily practice with three to five sun salutations, and then move into the other poses.

Within the sun salutations, the only posture that you hold for five breaths is downward facing dog. You will flow through all of the others, giving each one breath as indicated.

Inhale: Reach up and draw your palms together.

Exhale: Fold forward, bringing your palms to the floor. Your knees can be as bent as they need to be.

If you're practicing in a chair, fold forward over your legs and let your head hang loosely.

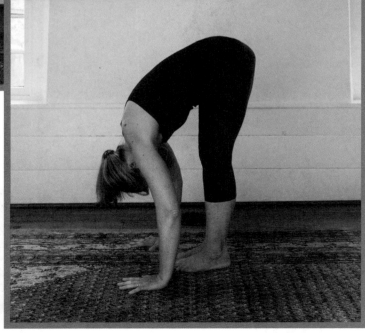

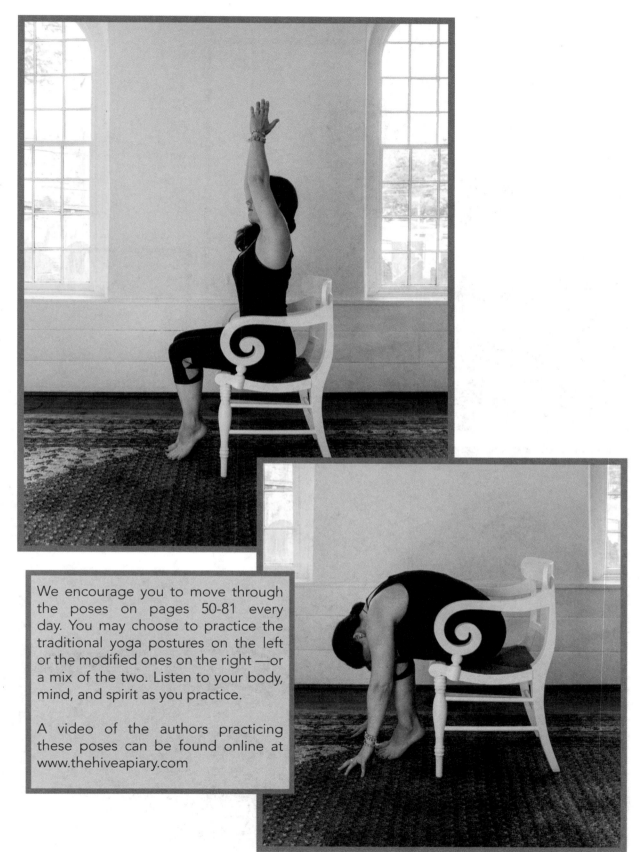

We encourage you to move through the poses on pages 50-81 every day. You may choose to practice the traditional yoga postures on the left or the modified ones on the right —or a mix of the two. Listen to your body, mind, and spirit as you practice.

A video of the authors practicing these poses can be found online at www.thehiveapiary.com

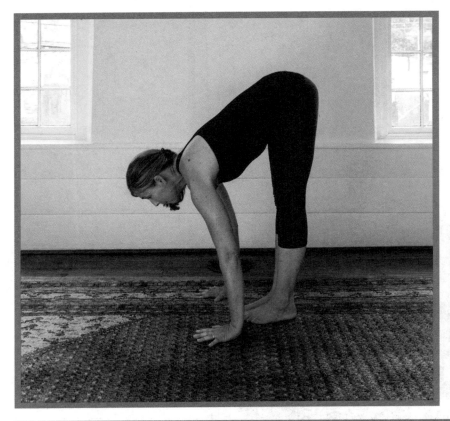

Inhale: Lift halfway, draw your shoulders away from your ears.

Exhale: Step backward to high plank. Your knees can be on or off the floor depending on your strength.

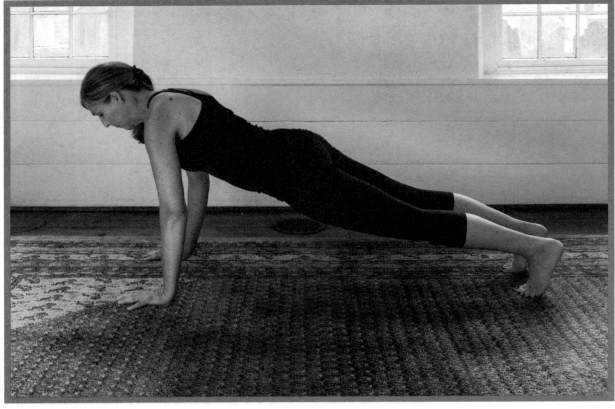

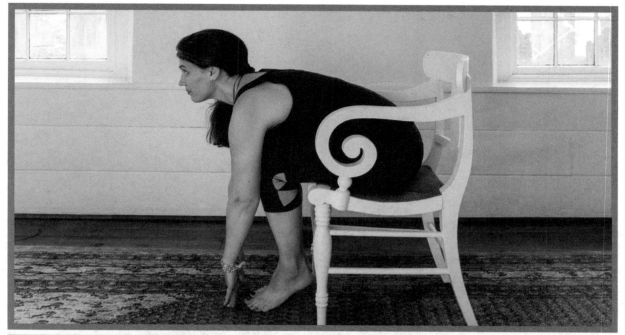

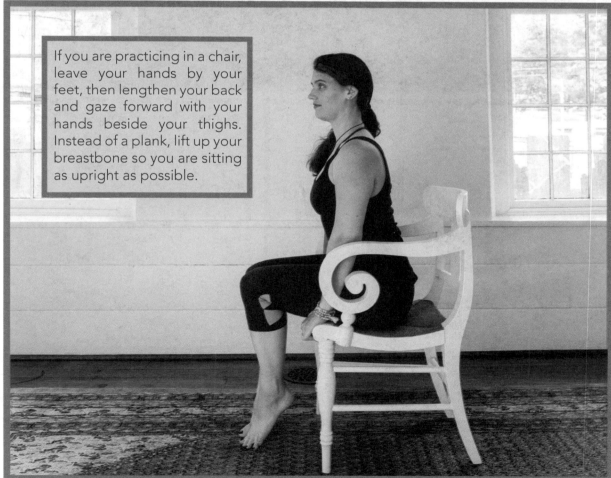

If you are practicing in a chair, leave your hands by your feet, then lengthen your back and gaze forward with your hands beside your thighs. Instead of a plank, lift up your breastbone so you are sitting as upright as possible.

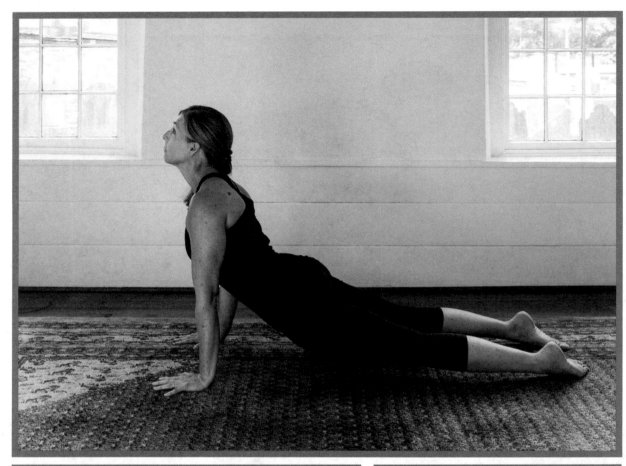

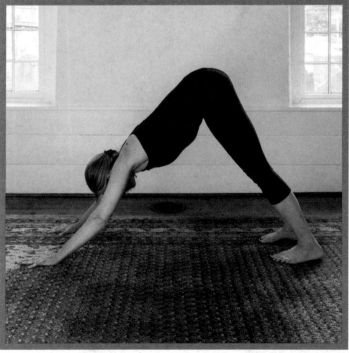

Inhale: Straighten your elbows to lift your chest into a gentle backbend. Press the tops of your feet into the floor. Your knees can be on or off the floor.

If you're practicing in a chair, continue to lift up through your chest as you drop your head back.

Exhale: Turn your toes under and lift your hips up, straightening your arms and pressing your hips back over feet. Drop your heels toward the floor. Stay here for 5 breaths.

If you're practicing in a chair, return to the previous posture and stay here, sitting tall, for 5 breaths.

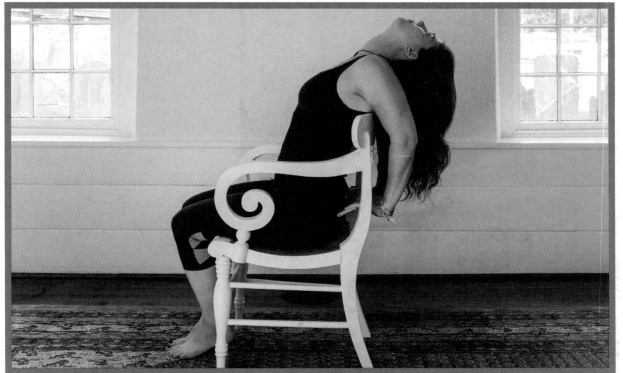

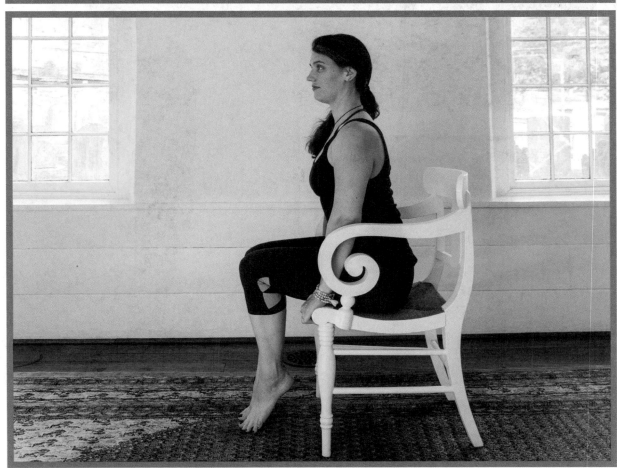

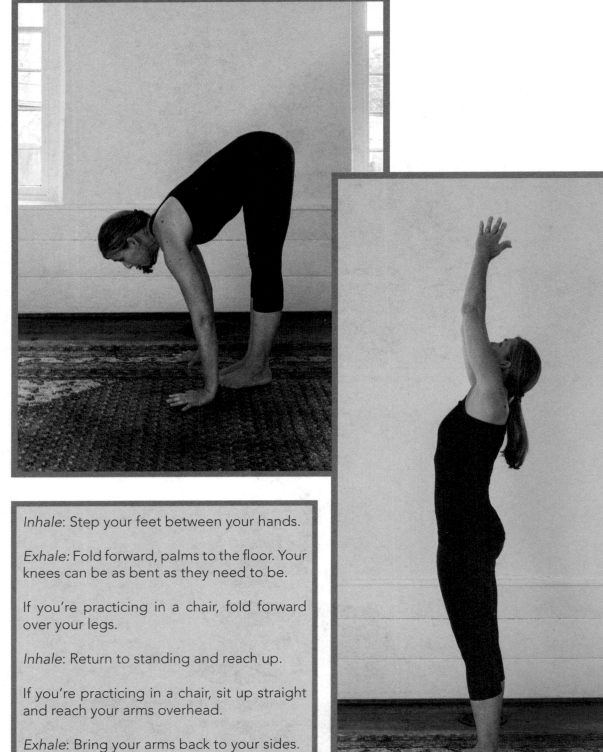

• Faith with a Twist

Inhale: Step your feet between your hands.

Exhale: Fold forward, palms to the floor. Your knees can be as bent as they need to be.

If you're practicing in a chair, fold forward over your legs.

Inhale: Return to standing and reach up.

If you're practicing in a chair, sit up straight and reach your arms overhead.

Exhale: Bring your arms back to your sides.

Repeat this series of movements 3-5 times.

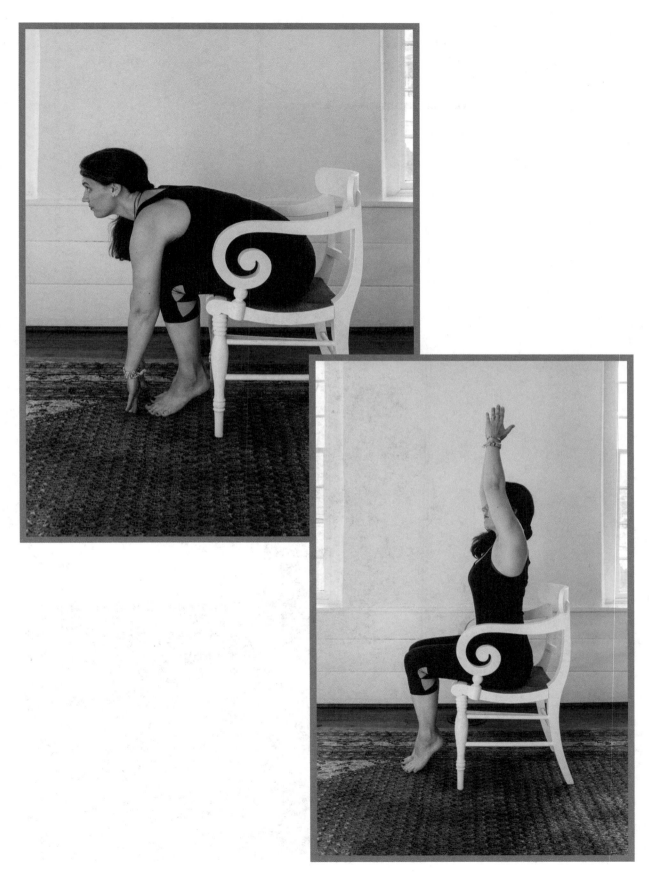

Padangusthasana
Standing Forward Fold

Inhale: Step your feet apart hip distance. Bring your hands to your hips. Gaze up.

Exhale: Fold forward and clasp your big toes. Your knees can be as bent as they need to be.

If you're practicing in a chair, fold forward and let your head hang loosely.

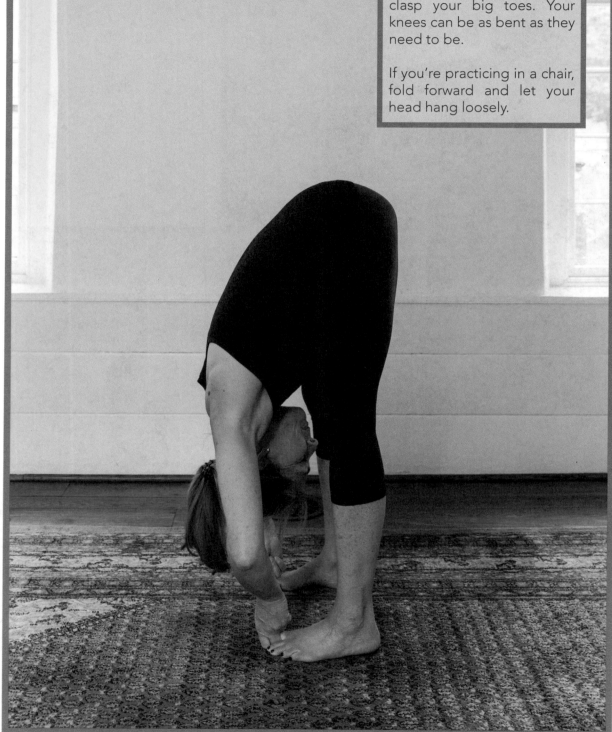

Inhale: Lift your chest and lengthen your back.

Exhale: Enter your forward fold by pulling your ribs toward your upper legs. Stay here for 5 breaths.

If you're practicing in a chair, clasp your toes and fold forward. Stay here for 5 breaths.

Inhale: Lift halfway.

Exhale: Bring your hands to your hips.

Inhale: Return to standing.

Exhale: Bring your arms to your sides and your feet together.

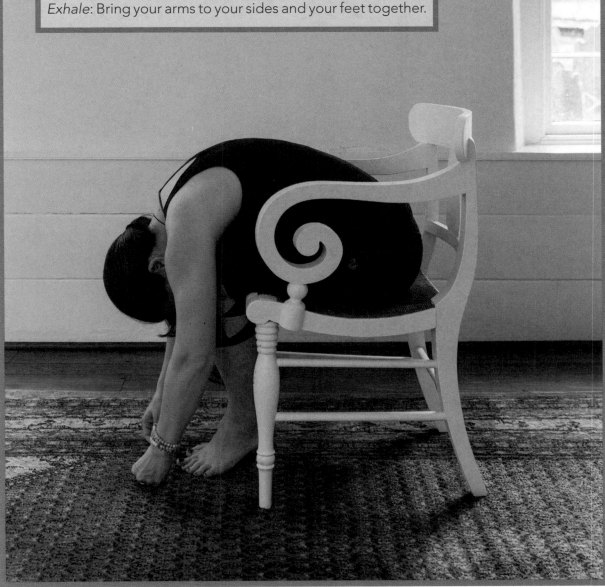

Trikonasana
Triangle Pose

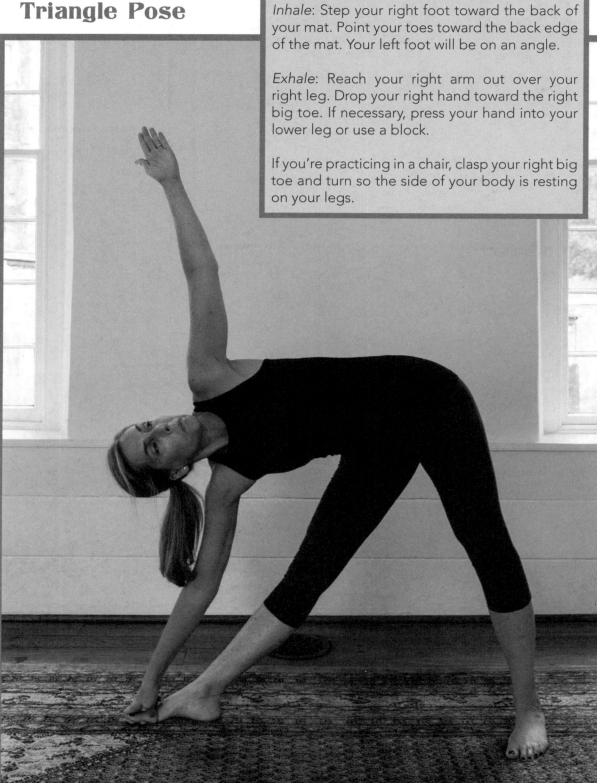

Inhale: Step your right foot toward the back of your mat. Point your toes toward the back edge of the mat. Your left foot will be on an angle.

Exhale: Reach your right arm out over your right leg. Drop your right hand toward the right big toe. If necessary, press your hand into your lower leg or use a block.

If you're practicing in a chair, clasp your right big toe and turn so the side of your body is resting on your legs.

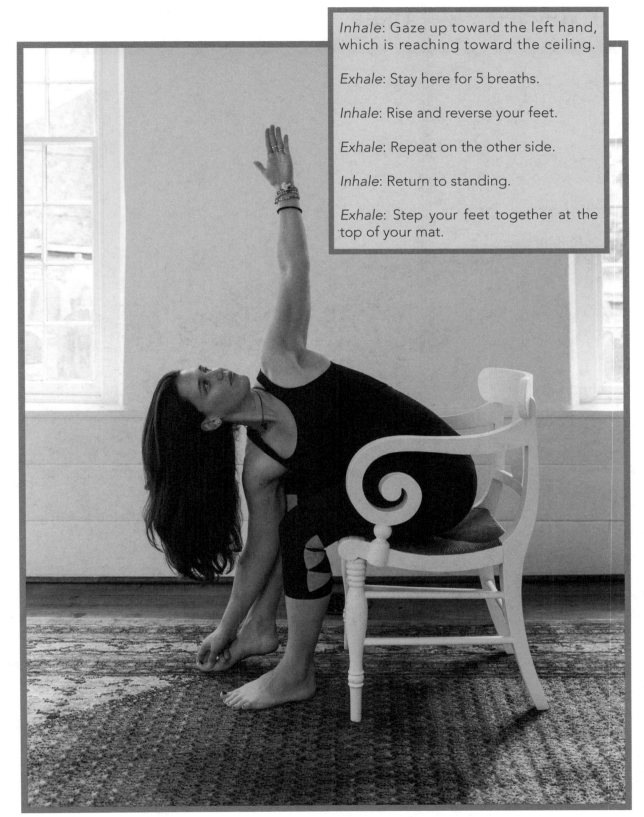

Inhale: Gaze up toward the left hand, which is reaching toward the ceiling.

Exhale: Stay here for 5 breaths.

Inhale: Rise and reverse your feet.

Exhale: Repeat on the other side.

Inhale: Return to standing.

Exhale: Step your feet together at the top of your mat.

Utthita Parsvakonasana
Extended Side Angle

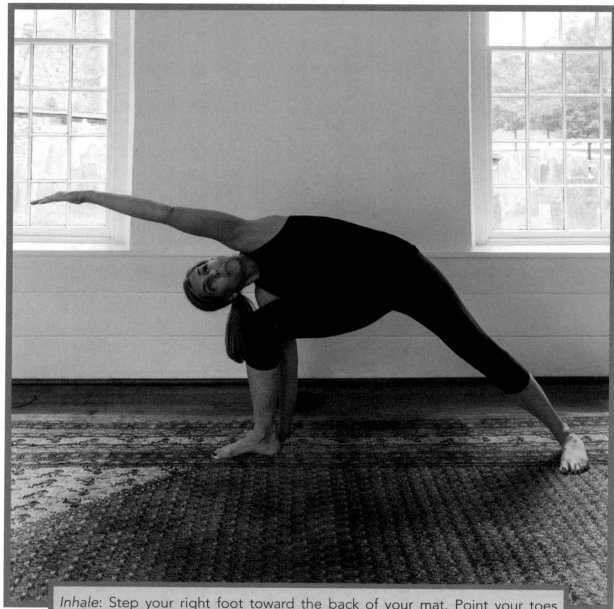

Inhale: Step your right foot toward the back of your mat. Point your toes toward the back edge of the mat. Your left foot will be at an angle.

Exhale: Bend your right knee. Be careful to keep your knee in line with your ankle. Rest your forearm on your bent leg or place your hand on the floor outside of your right foot.

If you need more support, feel free to rest your back knee on the floor or use a chair to aid your balance.

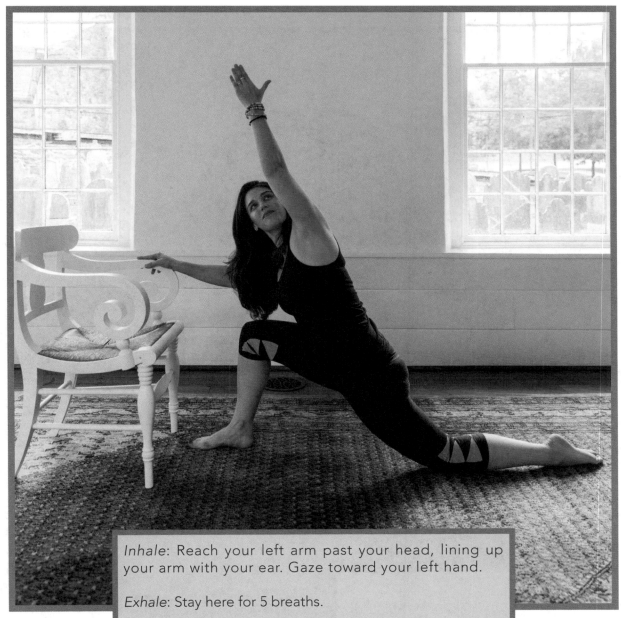

Inhale: Reach your left arm past your head, lining up your arm with your ear. Gaze toward your left hand.

Exhale: Stay here for 5 breaths.

Inhale: Rise and reverse your feet.

Exhale: Bend your left knee and repeat on the other side.

Inhale: Return to standing.

Exhale: Step your feet together at the top of your mat.

Prasarita Padottanasana D
Wide-Legged Forward Fold

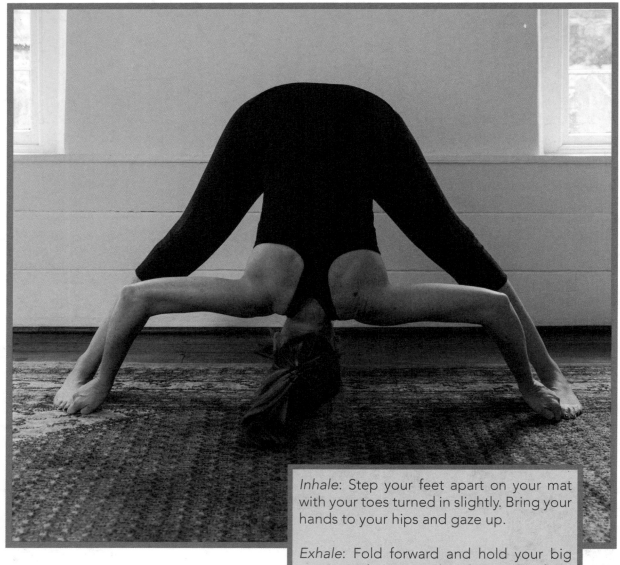

Inhale: Step your feet apart on your mat with your toes turned in slightly. Bring your hands to your hips and gaze up.

Exhale: Fold forward and hold your big toes or place your hands on the floor shoulder distance apart.

If you cannot reach the floor, your feet might be too close together. Try moving them apart until you can.

If touching the floor is not possible, feel free to use a chair for support and fold forward halfway.

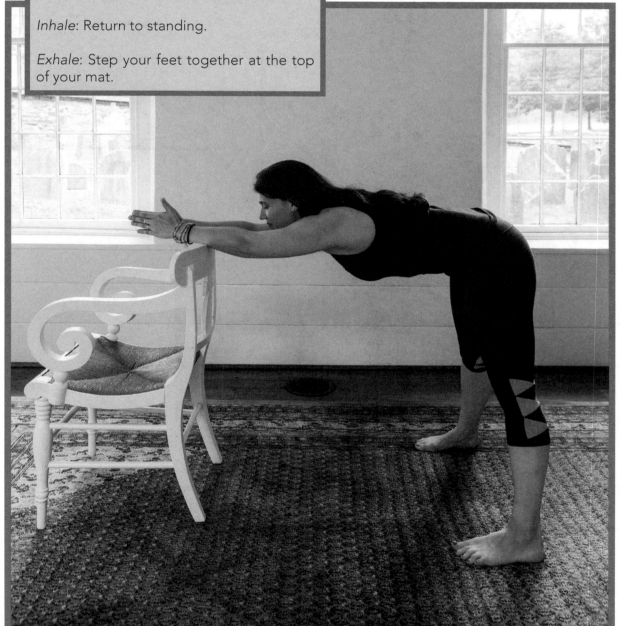

Inhale: Extend your breastbone away from your hips.

Exhale: Reach your head toward the floor. You may need to bend your elbows or even move your hands further back between your feet. Stay here for 5 breaths.

Inhale: Lift halfway.

Exhale: Bring your hands to your waist.

Inhale: Return to standing.

Exhale: Step your feet together at the top of your mat.

Vrkasana
Tree Pose

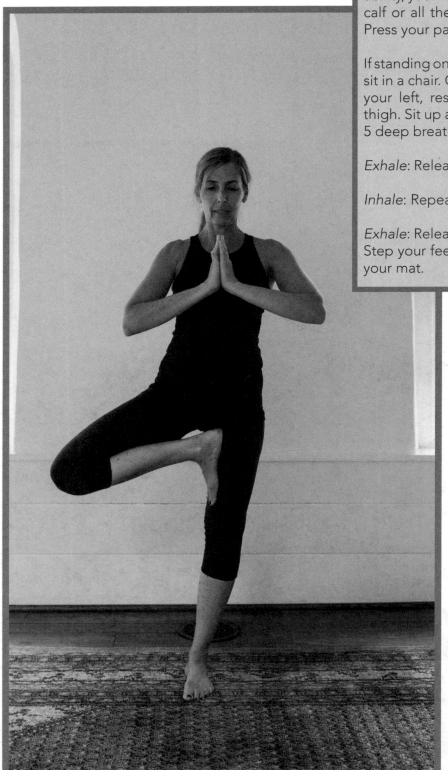

Inhale: Bring your right foot to your inner left leg. Depending on your ability, your foot will either be on your calf or all the way up on your thigh. Press your palms together.

If standing on one foot is not possible, sit in a chair. Cross your right leg over your left, resting the ankle on your thigh. Sit up as straight as you can for 5 deep breaths.

Exhale: Release your foot to the floor.

Inhale: Repeat on the other side.

Exhale: Release your foot to the floor. Step your feet together at the top of your mat.

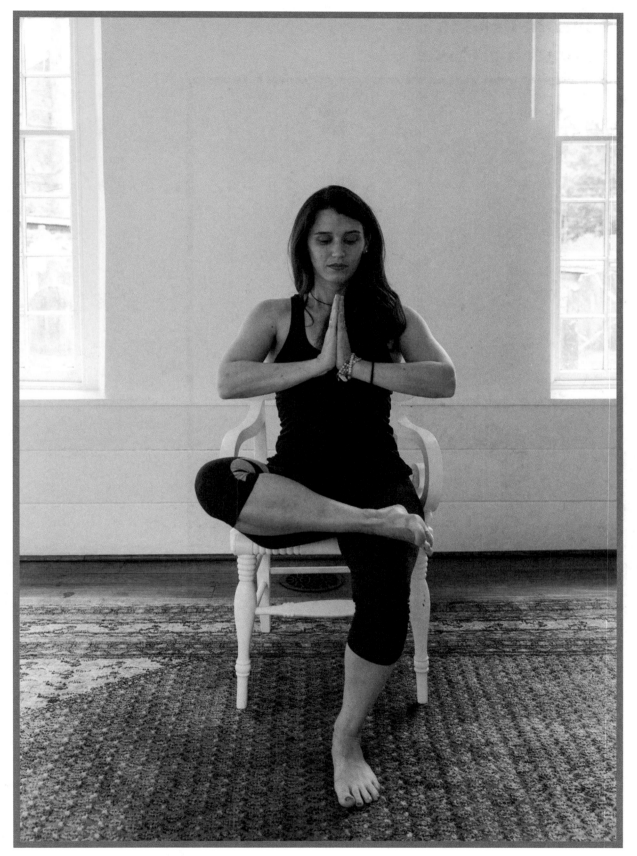

Virabhadrasana A
Warrior Pose

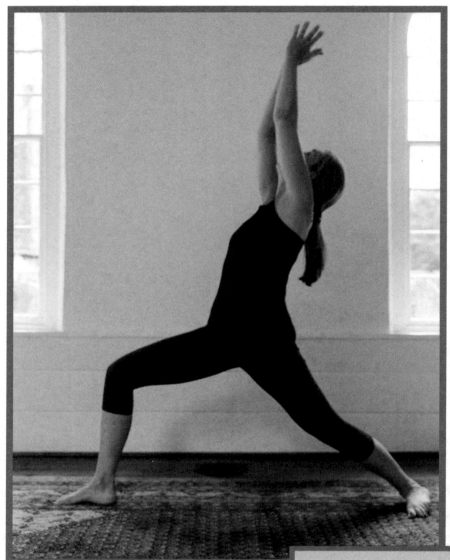

Inhale: Step your left foot toward the back of your mat. Line your heels up with each other. Your left toes will be on an angle.

Exhale: Bend your right knee and draw your hips to face the top of your mat.

Inhale: Reach up and press your palms together.

If you need support, feel free to use a chair.

Exhale: Stay here for 5 breaths.

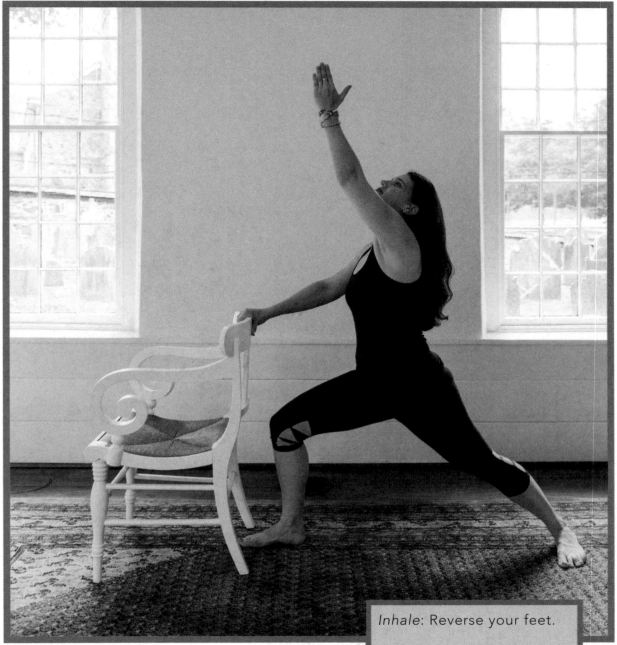

Inhale: Reverse your feet.

Exhale: Bend your left knee and repeat on the other side.

Inhale: Bring your hands to the mat and sit down.

Dandasana
Staff Pose

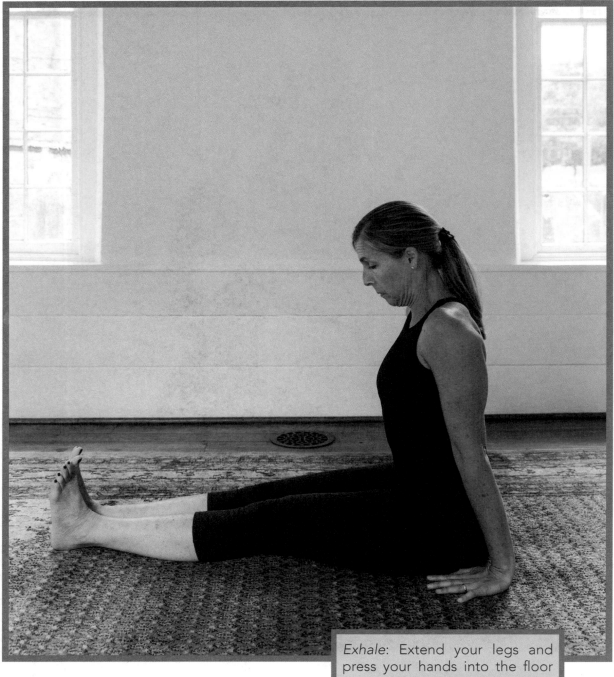

Exhale: Extend your legs and press your hands into the floor at your hips. Tuck your chin. Stay here for 5 breaths.

Paschimottanasana
Seated Forward Fold

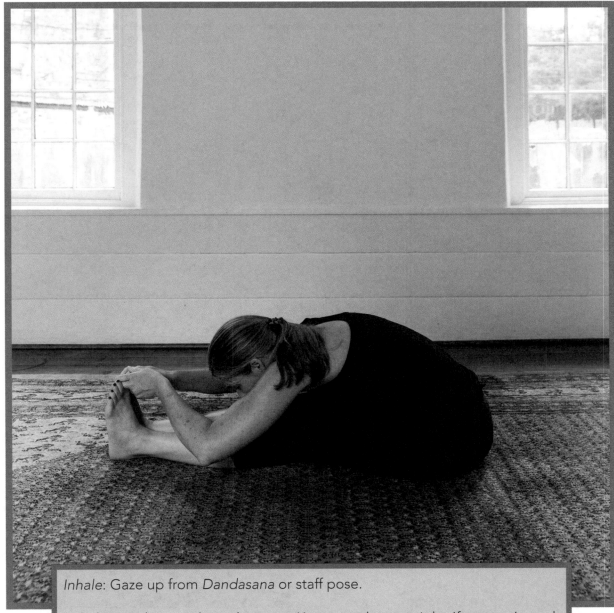

Inhale: Gaze up from *Dandasana* or staff pose.

Exhale: Reach toward your big toes. Keep your legs straight. If you can't reach your toes, hold on to your legs where you can. Stay here for 5 breaths.

Inhale: Lift your chest.

Exhale: Come all the way upright.

Janu Sirsasana
Head to Knee or Seated Tree Pose

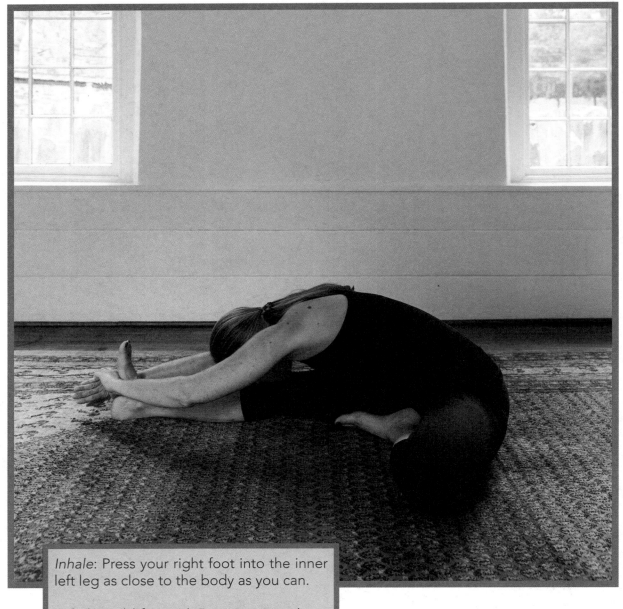

Inhale: Press your right foot into the inner left leg as close to the body as you can.

Exhale: Fold forward. Do not worry about getting your head to your leg. Keep your body as extended as possible. Stay here for 5 breaths.

If folding forward is too much, feel free to stay upright.

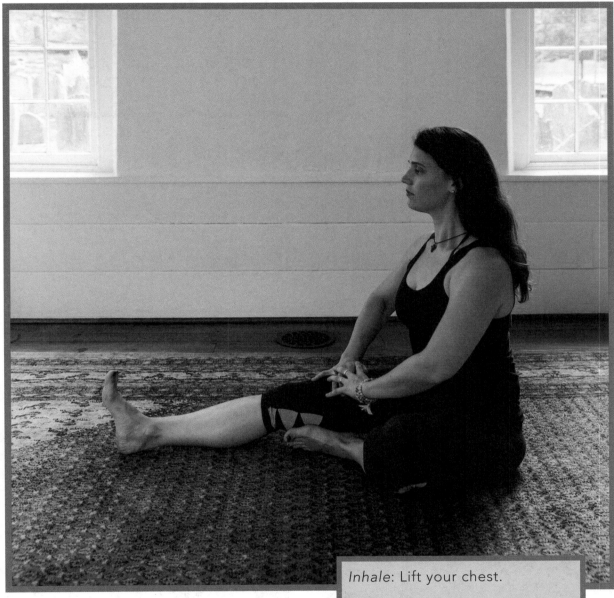

Inhale: Lift your chest.

Exhale: Come all the way upright and release the right leg.

Inhale: Repeat on the other side.

Exhale: Come all the way upright and extend your legs.

Marichyasana C
Seated Twist

Inhale: Bend your right leg. Your knee will point to the ceiling and your foot will be as close to your bottom as possible.

Exhale: Hug your bent leg with your left arm. Move into your twist and gaze over your right shoulder. If possible, you can move your left arm to your outer thigh and, pressing the upper arm into your outer leg, move into a deeper twist. Stay here for 5 breaths.

If you're practicing in a chair, sit upright as much as possible. Turn to gaze over your right shoulder. You can pull gently against the back of the chair to add intensity if it suits you.

Inhale: Face forward.

Exhale: Straighten your right leg.

Inhale: Repeat on the other side.

Exhale: Straighten your legs.

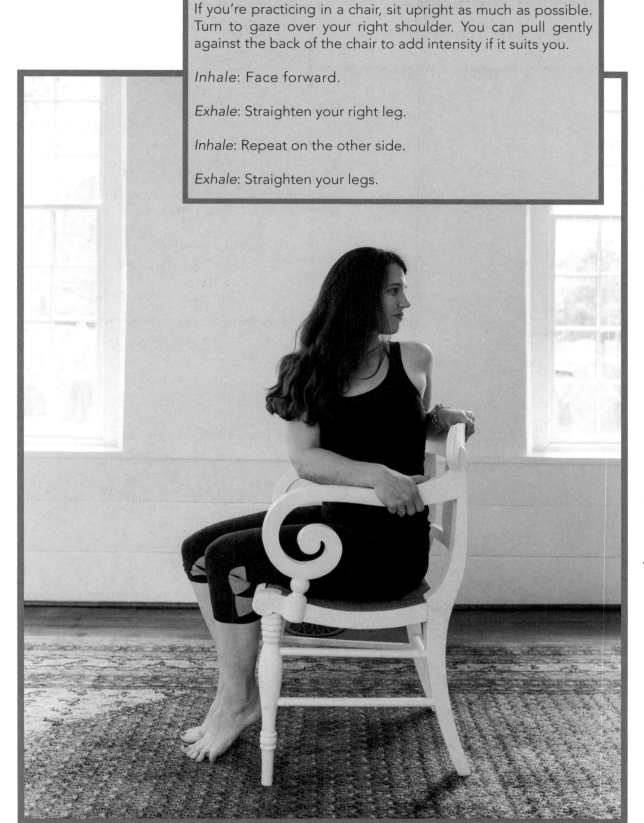

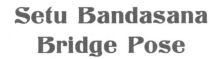

Setu Bandasana
Bridge Pose

Exhale: Lie down on your back.

Inhale: Bend both knees.

Exhale: Line your feet up with your hips.

If you're practicing in a chair, sit up as straight as possible. Without letting your ribs lower, drop your head back so that your upper back arches over the chair.

Inhale: Press your hips toward the ceiling. Stay here for 5 breaths.

Exhale: Lower your hips to the floor.

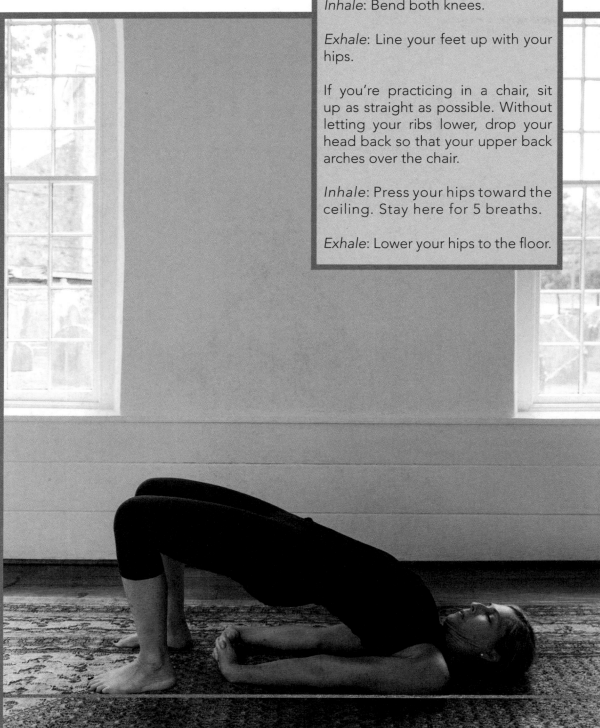

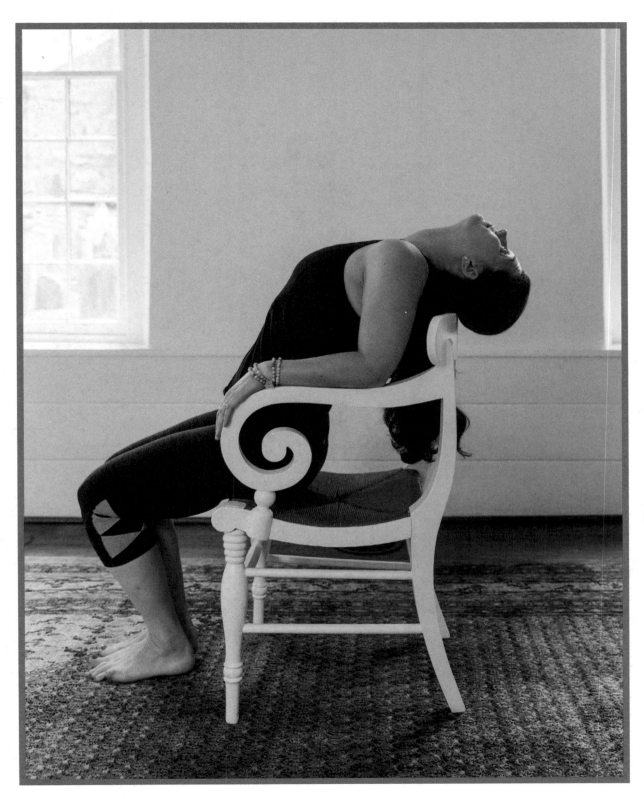

Viparita Karani
Legs Up the Wall Pose

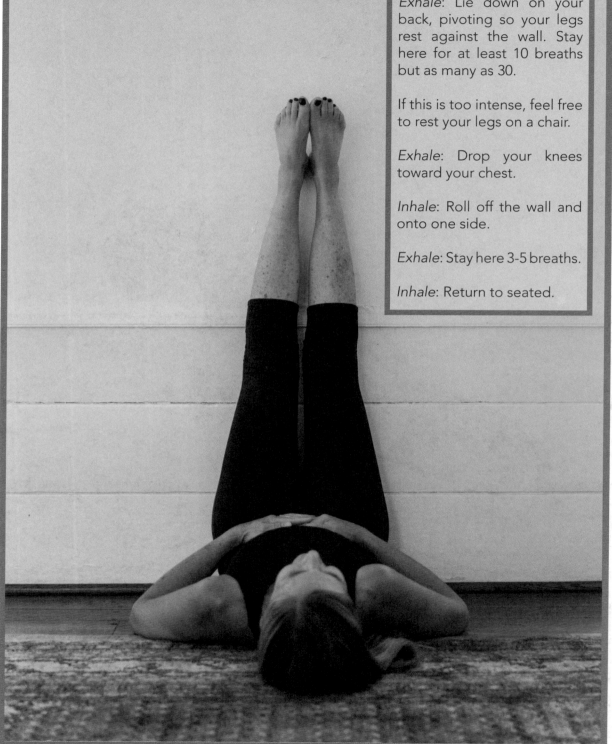

Inhale: Scoot over to a wall with your hips as close to the wall as possible.

Exhale: Lie down on your back, pivoting so your legs rest against the wall. Stay here for at least 10 breaths but as many as 30.

If this is too intense, feel free to rest your legs on a chair.

Exhale: Drop your knees toward your chest.

Inhale: Roll off the wall and onto one side.

Exhale: Stay here 3-5 breaths.

Inhale: Return to seated.

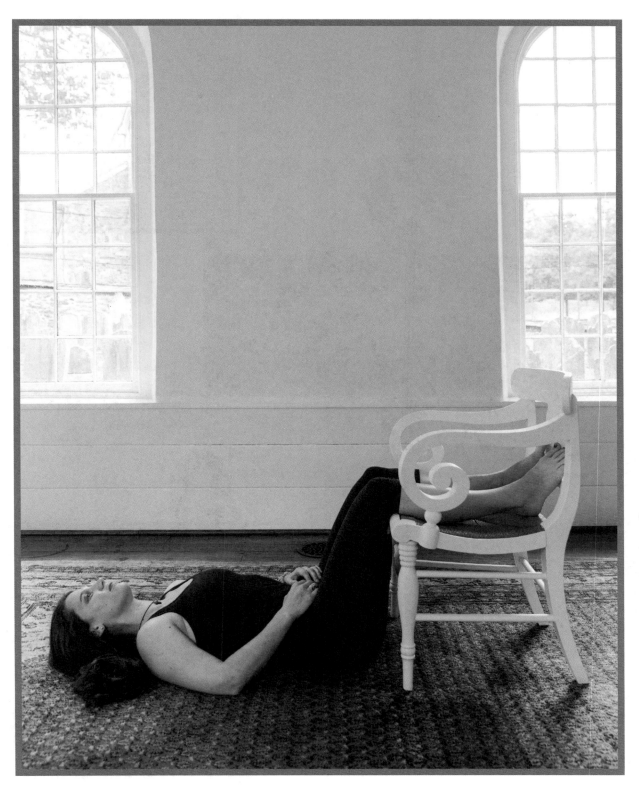

Padmasana
Lotus Pose

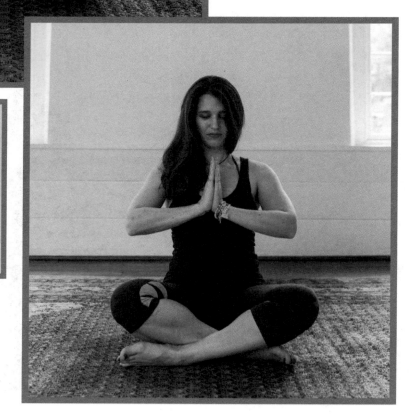

Inhale: Cross your legs.

To move into *padmasana*, draw the edge of your right foot into the crease where your left leg joins your body. Gently pull the left foot over the right lower leg and toward the body.

If this is too intense for your knees or ankles, find a comfortable cross-legged position or stay in your chair with your feet resting firmly on the floor.

Exhale: Rest the top of your hands on your knees, circling your index fingers and thumbs. Gently tuck your chin to your chest. Stay here for 10-20 breaths.

Inhale: Lift your head and release your hands.

Savasana
Corpse or Resting Pose

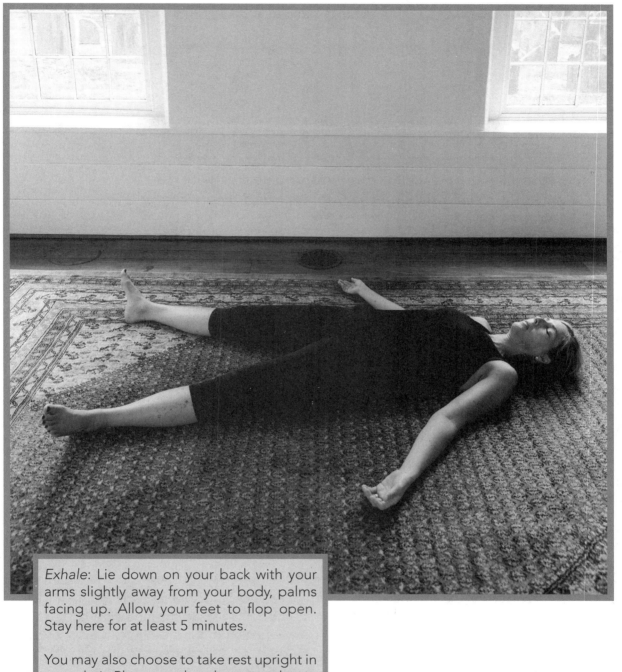

Exhale: Lie down on your back with your arms slightly away from your body, palms facing up. Allow your feet to flop open. Stay here for at least 5 minutes.

You may also choose to take rest upright in your chair. Place your hands on your knees with your palms facing up. Close your eyes.

Day 15
Aparigraha/Non-Possessiveness

Pray

> *Grant, most merciful Lord, to your faithful people pardon and peace, that they may be cleansed from all their sins, and serve you with a quiet mind; through Jesus Christ our Lord, who lives and reigns with you and the Holy Spirit, one God, forever and ever.* Amen.
> —*Lesser Feasts and Fasts*

Reflect

Today is our final day with both a focus on *aparigraha* as well as the group of *yamas*. We have journeyed through the difficult process of shedding old habits, patterns, and emotions in order to feel the lightness of the Holy Spirit. We have examined the reality of how much more effort it takes to cling onto things that no longer serve us, and we have practiced moving on. As you recall the original intention to rid yourself of habits or things that may separate you from God, use today to examine parts of your life on and off the mat that may need to change in order for you to create the space for new growth. These changes may be tangible (such as letting go of food habits or giving away excess clothing) or a spiritual thing (such as forgiving someone). What needs to move out so that something new can move in?

Practice

- Choose a closet or junk drawer or even your handbag or briefcase and clean it out. Enjoy parting with things that weigh you down, you don't need, or you are not using.
- Throw yourself a little "disappointment bonfire." Write down a disappointment (or several), place the paper in a safe container and then light it on fire. You can do the same type of thing by writing your disappointment on a coffee filter with a washable marker. Soak the filter in a bowl of water. You can also write your disappointment in sand, quiet yourself, and then smooth it over with a shovel or rake.
- Explore your experiences of *aparigraha* in your journal.

Change in Perspective

Inversions such as legs up the wall pose or, once your practice is more established, headstand (*sirsasana*), are intended to provide us with a much-needed change of perspective. It is amazing how difficult it is to adjust to being upside down. Your brain has to work doubly hard to figure out which way is up! Everything looks and feels different when you are upside down. The shift in perspective from a yoga inversion can leave you with a happy "hangover" of open-mindedness, a clear-eyed view of the world, and a willingness to leave behind old assumptions and ways of doing things. With all these benefits available to us, maybe it's not a bad idea to turn upside down at least once a day!

Pray

> *You bid your faithful people cleanse their hearts, and prepare with joy for the Paschal feast; that, fervent in prayer and in works of mercy, and renewed by your Word and Sacraments, they may come to the fullness of grace which you have prepared for those who love you.* Amen. —*The Book of Common Prayer*

Reflect

Practicing *sauca* (purity) means that we make a concentrated effort to keep ourselves clean, both on the outside (by bathing our bodies and keeping our clothing and homes clean) and on the inside (through *asana*, yoga's breathing exercises or *pranayama*, and eating a healthy diet).

When you think about *sauca*, imagine a lamp. If the glass of a lamp is dirty, the glow from the light inside cannot shine forth. A dirty lamp cannot fulfill its purpose of illuminating others. The same is true for us. Our yoga practices are building a light within each of us. This light becomes a beacon for others when we let our spirituality shine in our daily lives. As our practices deepen, the light grows stronger, eventually glowing enough that it draws others. The light that shines from us can lead others toward lives centered on intentional living and devotion.

However, if we do not care for our bodies and our environment, the light created by our yoga practices will be obscured. Others will not be able to see the light that is working in our lives.

We cannot hope to develop selfless care of others and the world around us until we have learned to care for ourselves. When we practice yoga, we learn to love ourselves, to respect our bodies, to be aware of our feelings and needs, and to feel and express gratitude for our bodies and our lives. As our practice with *sauca* deepens, the level of care that we are giving to our bodies expands further outward. Rather than developing into self-centeredness or preoccupation with appearance, *sauca* inevitably takes root and the world around us benefits.

Practice

On your mats today, consider where your body and space could use calming and purifying attention. Take time to make an inventory of your thoughts, feelings, and tensions. Does your mat need to be cleaned to remind you of making order in your world? Do your thoughts add to your practice, or are they distracting and need clarification? Does the space around you feel fresh and clean or do you need to set your surroundings in order?

You might identify hot-spot areas in your home, like an overflowing closet or a chaotic junk drawer that you can clean out. Or perhaps you take this process even further and ask how you can cleanse the world, such as joining a cleanup effort at a local park or watershed. However you express *sauca*, you will find yourself treating the world around you with heightened respect and tenderness.

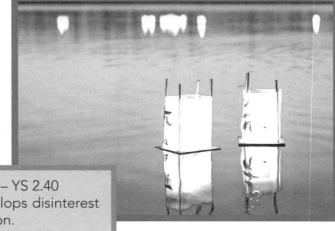

Saucatsvangajugupsa parairasmsargah. – YS 2.40
Cleanliness of the body and mind develops disinterest in contact with others for self-gratification.

Day 17
Sauca/Purity

Pray

Almighty God, to you all hearts are open, all desires known, and from you no secrets are hid: Cleanse the thoughts of our hearts by the inspiration of your Holy Spirit that we may perfectly love you, and worthily magnify your holy Name; through Christ our Lord. Amen. —The Book of Common Prayer

Reflect

In Paul's second letter to the Corinthians, he describes the way Jesus (who was pure from sin) came to free us from all impurities so that we might truly live in newness of life. Paul tells us that Jesus has come to reconcile us—the whole of ourselves—back to God and Jesus can do this amazing thing because of the purity of his love. Yet, we often think of this reconciliation as happening in the afterlife or sometime in the future. The joy of God's love for us, however, is that this is not a goal for us in the life to come but the true nature of our life in the here and now.

In order to live into this wonderful reality, we must first lay down burdens and impurities that plague our lives—we must confess our sins so that they will not stand in the way of our living as new creations. Today, consider making a confession (also known as Reconciliation of a Penitent) with your priest or in prayer with God. This is an especially appropriate practice in a season of self-examination. It is the invitation to a freeing spiritual purity that will let our true selves as unburdened children of God shine forth.

Once we have learned to love, respect, and listen to ourselves, it is perfectly natural to love, respect, and listen to others. Once we have learned to appreciate our bodies for all their uniqueness and quirkiness, for all they have to offer and despite all their shortcomings, it is much easier to appreciate others for their unique characteristics and quirks. In fact, we find ourselves feeling grateful for what others have to offer, despite their shortcomings. We learn to see others and ourselves as unique parts of an enormous, unfathomable whole. We learn to recognize the light of God shining in each and every one of us.

Practice

We can embrace *sauca* by how we approach our practice. Every breath we take is designed to purify the body and remove our toxins. The shape of many postures aid in digestion and help detoxify the organs. Holding an intense posture can clear out negative thoughts that may surface. These purification principles can be practiced on our mat to aid in our everyday life.

Eating and Drinking

You may have noticed that practicing yoga on a full stomach does not feel great. Doing so can give you heartburn, make you dizzy, or even make you feel nauseous. The rule of thumb is that you do not eat two hours before practicing, and you do not drink thirty minutes before practicing. This allows you to practice with an empty stomach, which makes you feel lighter and more focused as you move and breathe on your yoga mat.

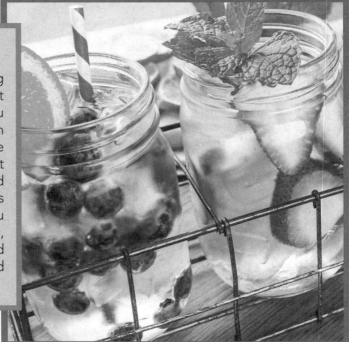

Day 18
Sauca/Purity

Pray

> Lord, make us instruments of your peace. Where there is hatred, let us sow love; where there is injury, pardon; where there is discord, union; where there is doubt, faith; where there is despair, hope; where there is darkness, light; where there is sadness, joy. Grant that we may not so much seek to be consoled as to console; to be understood as to understand; to be loved as to love. For it is in giving that we receive; it is in pardoning that we are pardoned; and it is in dying that we are born to eternal life. Amen.
> —The Book of Common Prayer

Reflect

In Jesus' time, the only way to be purified was to visit a temple to undertake ritualistic baths and offer sacrifices performed by an elite group of priests. An ordinary person could not hope to approach God without taking these measures, and you could be denied if you were deemed unlawful, shameful, or defiled. Jesus had strong words about this kind of thinking, reminding us that the act of purification is about being changed from the inside and has nothing to do with the external trappings that people tend to judge in one another. Jesus declares that we are all pure and worthy through him and we are all worthy to come to God. Our attention to purification then becomes a way of celebrating and honoring that love and closeness we have with God without judgment, shame, or need of an intermediary.

In the New Testament, Paul tells us our very bodies are temples of the Holy Spirit (1 Corinthians 6:19). When we make a choice to purify our bodies with clean food, deep practices, and rest, we honor the temples of the Holy Spirit. When we make a choice to purify our thoughts with prayer, meditation, and practice, we celebrate the closeness we have with God. When we make a choice to infuse our spirits with peace, forgiveness, and gratitude, we help the world become a holy place. How will you purify your world today?

Practice

Today we conclude our exploration of *sauca* with some suggestions on how you might engage this important *niyama* and build purity within and without.

- Spend some time learning about yogic purity rituals such as tongue sweepers and neti pots. Give one a try!
- Make sure the space that you practice in is calm and clutter free. Perhaps take this day to give it and your mat a thorough cleaning.
- Make an outline of a heart and divide it into sections representing the different feelings, emotions, or situations that are currently filling it. Use different colors to represent the way you feel about these things. Invite God into your heart to cleanse it from all impurities.
- Make sure to spend time concentrating on your breath and your twists in your practice. These are powerful cleansing agents for the body and soul.
- Again, consider making a confession with your priest or on your own with God to let go of the burden of sin and create the space for new life to spring forth.
- Explore your experiences with *sauca* in your journal.

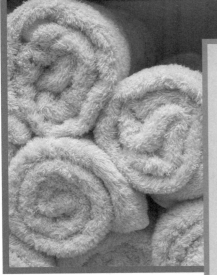

Hygiene

Traditionally, yoga is practiced after morning ablutions (in other words, after you have brushed your teeth and showered). Yoga's sister practice, *ayurveda* (the ancient Indian system of medicine) adds a few more cleansing rituals to our morning routine. In addition to cleaning our teeth, we also clean our tongue with a tongue scraper. This scraper can be made of stainless steel, but plastic ones are easily available in most local drug stores. We also wash our nasal passages with warm, salted water using a neti pot. These cleansing practices do a great deal to rid our body of irritants and bacteria each day. In doing so, many practitioners find they are less susceptible to minor illnesses such as the common cold and some even find their allergies become less severe.

Pray

Almighty Father, whose blessed Son before his passion prayed for his disciples that they might be one, as you and he are one: Grant that your Church, being bound together in love and obedience to you, may be united in one body by the one Spirit, that the world may believe in him whom you have sent, your Son Jesus Christ our Lord; who lives and reigns with you, in the unity of the Holy Spirit, one God, now and for ever. Amen. —The Book of Common Prayer

Reflect

Santosa (contentment) is one of the most powerful concepts in the philosophy of yoga. Practicing contentment shifts our perspective from one of need to one of abundance. *Santosa* teaches us to look around at our lives and be thankful for all we have—and for all our fulfilled needs. When we do, we feel contentment rather than dissatisfaction and unrest.

On our mats, we learn to be content with our "now." Each body is different because each body has its own individual life history that has brought it to its "now." There will always be people who are looser than us, or stronger than us, or taller or shorter or thinner than us. And, you know what? The same is true for all those people as well.

We have a choice. We can make ourselves crazy by looking around and judging ourselves against everybody in the room, in our town, or in the world. Or we can keep our eyes on our own mat. *Santosa* brings our focus back to us: here, now, today.

Life, as usual, turns out not to be too different from the little laboratories of our yoga mats. We find ourselves in situations that feel great and in situations that are really uncomfortable. That's life, right?

Santosa brings us face to face with an old, familiar test of faith. It's easy to rejoice in God's grace and gifts in times of abundance. The test comes when we're asked to maintain that same attitude of gratitude or reverence during difficult times. It's easy to hang out in our favorite *asana*, the one that makes us feel strong and flexible.

Can we do the same in a more challenging one? Can we maintain an attitude of gratitude when life is not going the way we wished it would go? When we try, we practice *santosa*.

Practice

We can start practicing contentment on our mats by exercising the willingness to stay in an uncomfortable *asana* and experience what it has to offer. We shift our focus away from our immediate discomfort to look toward opportunities to learn and grow. In other words, we breathe instead of react. Our practice is a perfect place to notice how content we are or are not. Can you be content even when you are straining to hold a difficult pose? When you are in your final pose, let your body rest in peaceful contentment knowing that no matter what happened in your practice today, you have been given gifts that can carry you until you return again.

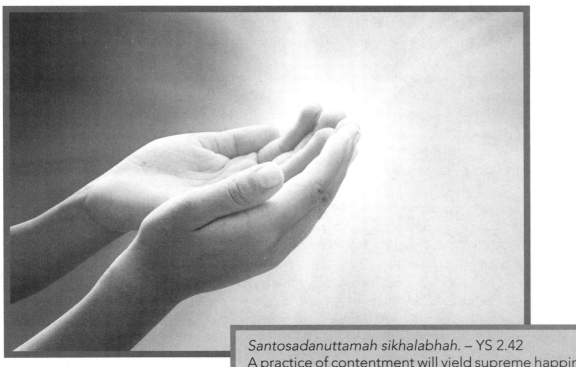

Santosadanuttamah sikhalabhah. – YS 2.42
A practice of contentment will yield supreme happiness.

Day 20
Santosa/Contentment

Pray

> *Grant us, O Lord our Strength, a true love of your holy Name; so that, trusting in your grace, we may fear no earthly evil, nor fix our hearts on earthly goods, but may rejoice in your full salvation; through Jesus Christ our Lord, who lives and reigns with you and the Holy Spirit, one God, for ever and ever.* Amen.
> *—Lesser Feasts and Fasts*

Reflect

As we contemplate the nature of *santosa*, let us turn to Jesus who is often called our comforter and the Prince of Peace. Jesus is our center of joy and peace, the source of all calmness, making him the one who can teach our hearts to dwell in contentment.

In the Gospel of John, Jesus describes himself as the good shepherd who can so put his sheep at ease that even the sound of his voice offers them contentment and guidance to pastures of tranquility. He says, "Very truly, I tell you, I am the gate for the sheep. All who came before me are thieves and bandits, but the sheep did not listen to them. I am the gate. Whoever enters by me will be saved, and will come in and go out and find pasture" (John 10:7-9).

This kind of love and guidance is truly an invitation to contentment: If we but follow the voice of the God who loves us, then whether we "come in or go out," we will be content and find what we need to achieve *santosa*.

When we are able to practice contentment, we not only gain a peace, but also we discover something unshakable—the knowledge that we are not alone and that no matter the hardships that might befall us, God is with us. Gratitude like that is powerful.

Practice

This passage from the Gospel of John offers a wonderful *mantra* (a phrase to help keep focus) during meditative breathing. Concentrate on knowing that God gives us all that we need. Begin by taking a deep breath and repeating the phrase, "Come in," and then exhale saying "And go out." Pause, and then add the final part of the phrase: "And find pasture." God carries us in every moment just as our breath flows in and out of our bodies. This exercise helps us to remember that we are never separated from the life-giving flow of the Spirit.

Corpse or Resting Pose

It can be tempting to skip right over the last posture of our practice, *savasana* (corpse pose or resting pose). We invite you to resist that temptation and commit to a longer stay in this posture than feels natural—up to ten minutes! During the rest at the end of practice, several things are happening physically. Your body is absorbing all the work it just did. Your joints and muscles are adjusting to their new positions. Your heart and breathing rates are slowing down from their faster practice paces. If you built up some internal heat, your body is using this time to cool down. If you were lucky enough to break a sweat, let the perspiration dry on your skin. It is said to contain minerals that will give you a youthful glow!

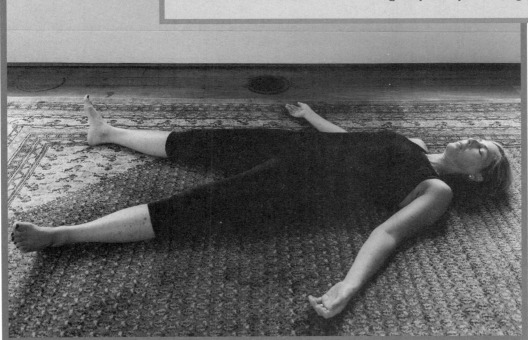

Day 21
Santosa/Contentment

Pray

Most loving Father, whose will it is for us to give thanks for all things, to fear nothing but the loss of you, and to cast all our care on you who care for us: Preserve us from faithless fears and worldly anxieties, that no clouds of this mortal life may hide from us the light of that love which is immortal, and which you have manifested to us in your Son Jesus Christ our Lord; who lives and reigns with you, in the unity of the Holy Spirit, one God, now and forever. Amen.
—*The Book of Common Prayer*

Reflect

At times, we struggle with being content because we fail to notice all the messages of love that surround us and instead respond to the constant cry to desire more. Think back to an "Aha!" moment when you recognized something you were truly grateful for. Describe that feeling in your journal.

Practice

As we conclude our exploration of *santosa*, let us invite God into every moment, remembering that the heart of contentment can be found in joy and gratitude. Here are some suggestions:

- Start a gratitude journal. Today's entry could be a list of all the things and people you are grateful for in your life.
- Think of an object that makes you feel jealous or envious. See it clearly. Ask yourself why you want it. Would your life really be better if you had it? Look at your life without this object and see all the ways your life is full without it. This is a great exercise to do in writing.
- Explore your own experiences with *santosa* in your journal.

How often do you need to practice?

Ashtanga yoga, which is the kind of yoga that we practice, prescribes practice six days a week with a sabbath day of rest. Even so, it is a good idea to start slowly and build up gradually. While many students come to class once or twice a week, we encourage you to follow our favorite yoga rule of thumb: "A little yoga a lot is better than a lot of yoga a little." In short, invite yourself to a daily practice: Do what feels right to you, and you will be doing it exactly right.

Day 22
Tapas/Self-Discipline

Pray

> *O God, by whom the meek are guided in judgment, and light rises up in darkness for the godly: Grant us, in all our doubts and uncertainties, the grace to ask what you would have us to do, that the Spirit of wisdom may save us from all false choices, and that in your light we may see light, and in your straight path may not stumble; through Jesus Christ our Lord.* Amen.
> *—The Book of Common Prayer*

Reflect

We have all made commitments because we felt we should do something rather than because we cared deeply about the cause. When we're dashing through our days feeling overwhelmed and frantic, it is easy to cancel a "should." We are much more likely to squeeze in time for something we care about. The principle of *tapas* is commitment with passion.

In our yoga practices, *tapas* raises the old question, "Which came first: the chicken or the egg?" Only, this time we're asking, "Which comes first: dedication or passion?" The reality is that *tapas* builds as our practice builds. Dedication and passion support one another.

You have probably noticed that yoga is not easy. While we may have a posture or two that are easy for us, the practice as a whole is hard. It asks a lot of us: strength, flexibility, humility, and courage.

In *asana* practice, we learn that we cannot reap the benefits of a posture if we're not working in the posture. While we need to be comfortable enough in each posture so that we can maintain long, slow, even breaths, we simply cannot be lazy. In fact, Pattabhi Jois, the creator of *ashtanga* yoga, was fond of saying that yoga is for everybody—strong, weak, healthy, and sick. Only lazy people cannot do yoga. Just as you can't be lazy in yoga postures, you can't be lazy in life either. In *Meditations on the Mat*, Rolf Gates describes *tapas* as more than the willingness to work hard in practice but rather a principle rooted in genuine desire. Our desire for spiritual health, stronger bodies, and focused minds will give us consistency in our practice. We will have good days and bad days, days when the spirit is willing, but the flesh is weak, and days when the opposite is the case. Building a steady, committed practice, one that will last for years, requires a passionate desire to know more, grow more, and develop more.

Practice

Our yoga practice can help us bring our passion to the foreground as we observe the amount of work we are willing to put into a posture. It takes passion to come to our mats and be fully present, to give our all to our breath, our count, our strength, and our goals without losing focus on what truly matters—our union with the Spirit. Be passionate today as you gain the desire for *tapas*. You should be sweaty by the end of today's practice!

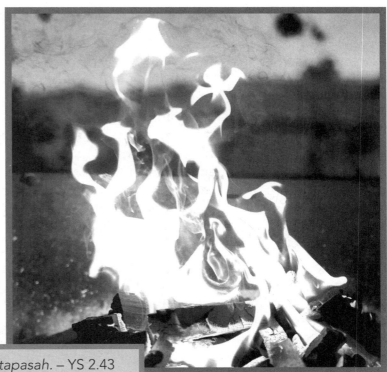

Kayendriyasiddhirasuddhiksayat tapasah. – YS 2.43
When we practice self-discipline, impurities are destroyed, and we gain spiritual strength.

Day 23
Tapas/Self-Discipline

Pray

O God, with you is the well of life, and in your light we see light: Quench our thirst with living water, and flood our darkened minds with heavenly light; through Jesus Christ our Lord, who lives and reigns with you and the Holy Spirit, one God, for ever and ever. Amen.
—Lesser Feasts and Fasts

Reflect

We often think of Jesus as being calm and peaceful. Yet, he was the very epitome of *tapas*! Take this passage from the Gospel of John: "The Passover of the Jews was near, and Jesus went up to Jerusalem. In the temple he found people selling cattle, sheep, and doves, and the money changers seated at their tables. Making a whip of cords, he drove all of them out of the temple, both the sheep and the cattle. He also poured out the coins of the money changers and overturned their tables. He told those who were selling the doves, 'Take these things out of here! Stop making my Father's house a marketplace!' His disciples remembered that it was written, 'Zeal for your house will consume me'" (John 2:13-17).

We see here a passionate Jesus who is focused and determined in his quest for the moral integrity of the worship of God. Jesus, who is indeed the Prince of Peace, was also the disruptor of false peace. After all, people who "keep the peace" rarely get crucified. Nor do they change the world. When it comes to standing up for justice, there can be no weakness of spirit.

The zeal Jesus displayed should show up in own lives. We will never know true peace until we are ready to stand up for what is true and pure. Only with that kind of *tapas* will we know the fire of the Holy Spirit.

Practice

In your prayers and on your mat today, ask that same Spirit to join you in your quest for a zealous love of God and let it consume you in a way that will bring true peace to your life.

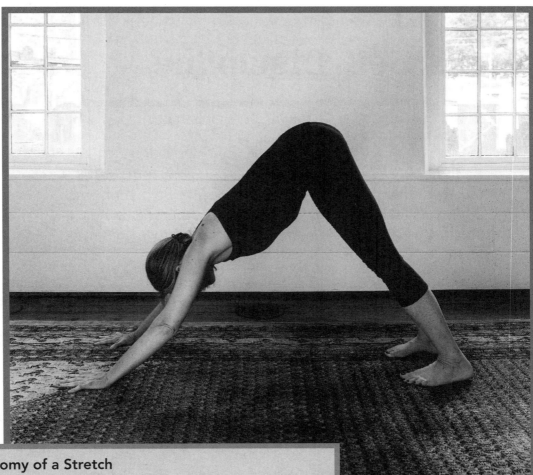

The Anatomy of a Stretch

By now you have noticed that something happens when you hold each yoga posture for five deep breaths. (These five breaths should take about twenty-five seconds. They are much longer, slower, and deeper than your regular breathing). In the first breath or two, you may feel as if you've hit a wall, that you simply cannot go any further into the posture. This feeling is called resistance. Your muscle has moved to the end of its comfortable range of motion. When we stay at this edge and keep breathing, the resistance dissolves a little. This is called a release and often happens during the third or fourth breath. While you're on the yoga mat, your job is to move mindfully—to stretch—into this newly available space. Over time and with practice, this new range of motion will become your norm, and you will be able to stretch past it as you develop more flexibility.

Day 24
Tapas/Self-Discipline

Pray

I will try this day to live a simple, sincere, and serene life, repelling promptly every thought of discontent, anxiety, discouragement, impurity, and self-seeking; cultivating cheerfulness, magnanimity, charity, and the habit of holy silence; exercising economy in expenditure, generosity in giving, carefulness in conversation, diligence in appointed service, fidelity to every trust, and a childlike faith in God.

In particular I will try to be faithful in those habits of prayer, work, study, physical exercise, eating, and sleep, which I believe the Holy Spirit has shown me to be right. And as I cannot in my own strength do this, nor even with a hope of success attempt it, I look to thee, O Lord God my Father, in Jesus my Savior, and ask for the gift of the Holy Spirit. Amen.
—A Morning Resolve, Forward Day by Day

Reflect

As we come to the last day of our exploration of *tapas*, let us remember that we are called to find areas in our life, on and off the mat, that can be infused with a passion for God and for peace. Our prayer for the day speaks of a kind of *tapas*—a zeal and resolve to shape our lives in such a way that all our actions point to our goal of following the Holy Spirit. In what ways can you live into that prayer today? How can you bring *tapas* to your lived-out faith?

Practice

- On your mat today, find poses that can help you express the balance between passion and peace. For example, in warrior (pages 66-67), try to move into your lunge as deep as you can and hold it for 10 counts. Even as you bring more effort to the physical aspect of the pose, try to remain calm. Become a peaceful warrior.
- Take some time to ask God for clarity of mind and spirit to help you see what parts of your life need the touch of true peace. Where is there injustice? Where is there need for vigilance? Where is there a need to invite passion?
- Make sure that you are coming to your mat with vigor. Pay particular attention to your breath, as it is the bellows of your inner fire.

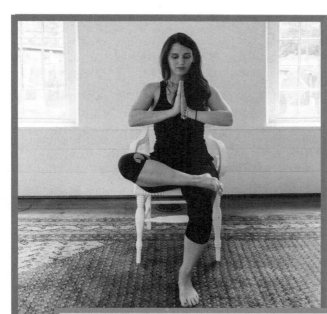

Mental Benefits of Yoga

Yoga is good for the body and the spirit, but it is also very good for the mind. As we draw our awareness back to our alignment and our breath, we are training ourselves to have better focus. This benefits us in everything we do: our work, hobbies, sports, and even relaxation. Yoga helps us to step into the driver's seat of our minds. On average, a person thinks 60,000 thoughts a day, many of which take us away from the present moment and into worry, anticipation, regret, or recollection. A mindful practice such as yoga helps us choose to be present to what is happening right here and right now.

Day 25
Svadhyaya/Self-Study

Pray

Holy God, your knowledge of me exceeds what I grasp or see in any moment; you know me better than I know myself. Now, help me to trust in your mercy, to see myself in the light of your holiness, and grant me the grace that I may have true contrition, make an honest confession, and find in you forgiveness and perfect remission. Amen. —Saint Augustine's Prayer Book

Reflect

Svadhyaya's typical translation from Sanskrit to English reveals its two-pronged meaning. We usually translate *svadhyaya* as "the education of the self or self-study." Can you see the two veins of meaning? When we educate ourselves, we're learning from others. When we practice self-study, we're learning from ourselves.

It is our duty to listen and learn from our teachers, and then to go deeper into whatever subject we are learning. The teacher cannot push; he or she can only guide. *Svadhyaya* asks us to be the driver in our education.

The other half of *svadhyaya* is study of the self. While the first form of study happens primarily off our mats, we can easily begin this portion of the practice on our mats. By focusing on our reactions, habits, preferences, aversions, assumptions, and areas of ignorance on our mats, we can begin to see those same habits and practices in our lives off our mats. We might recognize how quickly we jump to conclusions when faced with challenges or when we recall how we assumed a posture was out of our reach without even trying it. We might discover the same work ethic in our day-to-day lives that we exhibited when we were able to hold a taxing pose for five full breaths.

As we come to know ourselves intimately, we discover the divinity at our core. When self-study has brought us to the place where we truly know God is within us just as we are within God, we also come to know that the same is true for everyone else. By deepening our understanding of ourselves, we come to understand others. The understanding we gain opens the way to love.

Practice

Today as you practice, think of yourself as student and teacher. Allow yourself to play both roles with passion. What can you teach yourself? What can you learn from yourself? How do these things translate into your life once you roll up your yoga mat?

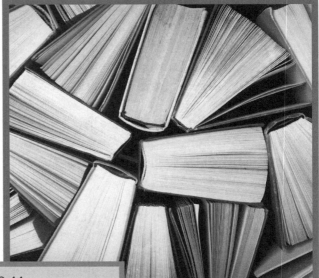

Svadhyayadisthadevatasamprayogah. – YS 2.44
When we embrace self-study, we immerse ourselves in God.

Day 26
Svadhyaya/Self-Study

Pray

> *Blessed Lord, who caused all holy Scriptures to be written for our learning: Grant us so to hear them, read, mark, learn, and inwardly digest them, that we may embrace and ever hold fast the blessed hope of everlasting life, which you have given us in our Savior Jesus Christ; who lives and reigns with you and the Holy Spirit, one God, for ever and ever.* Amen.
> —*The Book of Common Prayer*

Reflect

Jesus was always offering moments of *svadhyaya* to his disciples. The gospels are full of Jesus teaching and leading his followers to places of transformation and inner wisdom, if they would but heed his lessons.

In the Gospel of Luke, the apostles come to Jesus, asking for instruction in how to pray. "He said to them, 'When you pray, say: Father, hallowed be your name. Your kingdom come. Give us each day our daily bread. And forgive us our sins, for we ourselves forgive everyone indebted to us. And do not bring us to the time of trial'" (Luke 11:2-4).

Notice how Jesus offers opportunities for *svadhyaya* to his followers.

First, he gives them the example of praying himself. A true teacher only earns the right to teach through his or her own dedication and wisdom to continued learning and growth. Jesus shows his mark as a true teacher and person of faith by being attentive to his own spiritual life, and his disciples take notice.

Second, he is open to their questions and indeed teaches them how to pray. Finally, Jesus offers a prayer rich and multilayered. Even its poetic brevity is a thing of beauty. The disciples are able to easily memorize the prayer so that they will be able to gain lessons from it in years to come.

Our yoga practice is designed to offer similar moments of clarity. Through practice, God gives us the space to follow the example of wise spiritual leaders.

We are able to ask questions about our life and find answers through practice. And finally, we have a series of postures that we can memorize so we can have this practice any time and in any place.

Practice

Today, come to your practice with the same mindset that the disciples did as they approached Jesus. Ask your practice to teach you about yourself and about peace. Like the Lord's Prayer, your practice will be there for you over and over with wisdom and new lessons every time you come to the mat.

Different Kinds of Yoga

The tree of yoga has many branches. The series of practices in this book is based on *ashtanga* yoga. *Ashtanga* is a vigorous, flowing style of yoga for which the breath and its synchronization with the movement of the body is of the highest importance. Other styles of yoga abound and the following list is far from exhaustive. *Iyengar* yoga is a precise practice that is focused on alignment. *Yin* yoga has a very slow pace where you hold each posture for minutes at a time. *Vinyasa* yoga is a flowing style of yoga found in many health and fitness clubs. *Bikram* yoga is a set series of twenty-six postures taught in a heated room. Power yoga often refers to a more vigorous *vinyasa* flow class. Restorative yoga is a quiet practice designed to soothe nerves and settle the mind.

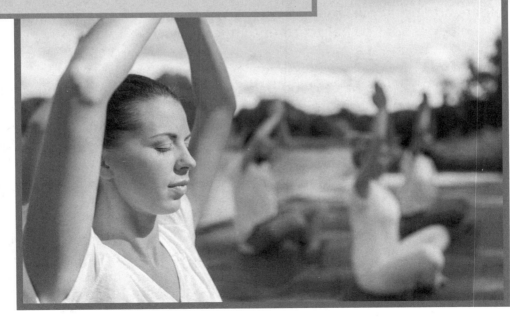

Pray

Lord, we pray that your grace may always precede and follow us, that we may continually be given to good works; through Jesus Christ our Lord, who lives and reigns with you and the Holy Spirit, one God, now and forever. Amen. —The Book of Common Prayer

Reflect

In our Western culture, people often look outside themselves for expert opinions on all matters. However, this leaves behind the internal wisdom of our own souls and bodies. How do you know when you really "know" something? Is it a feeling in your gut? Does your heart ring out? Do you have butterflies in your stomach? These are all ways that our bodies can hold wisdom that cannot be given to us from the outside. How can you learn to trust the messages of your inner guru?

Practice

As we conclude our discussion of *svadhyaya*, remember that these thirty days are an intense time of self-study. We are called to use this time to grow in our understanding of our true nature and to then learn from our loving God. Here are some suggestions to help further that journey.

- If you do not have a yoga teacher or a spiritual director, consider finding one you trust who has a good balance of teaching styles for you. Guides along the way are the best form of learning about ourselves.
- Start (or continue) journaling, even if you write just a few lines every day. This will help you notice patterns or see transformation. This practice can be especially useful during prayer time.
- Consider spending more time in scripture study today. Perhaps choose an entire gospel to read at one sitting. This exercise will bring you closer to the desires and will of our ultimate teacher, Jesus.
- Try one new thing today that you have never done before. Maybe it's a new posture on your mat. Maybe it's a new kind of food. Maybe you talk to a new person on the street. Whatever you try, notice what you learn about yourself.

Gear

Yoga requires very little in terms of equipment. Most importantly, you will need a yoga mat. Choosing a mat is a personal decision. Prices can range widely. Until you know what you like and what you don't, we suggest spending $15 to $20 for a perfectly reasonable first mat. Once you have committed to a practice, you can choose a long-term (and more expensive) mat. You can choose a mat based on thickness, texture, size (longer or wider), and the material (organic and biodegradable or man-made). You will also want to consider whether or not your hands and feet sweat a lot; certain mats get slippery. Be sure to choose a color that makes you smile!

Day 28
Isvara Pranidhana/Devotion to God

Pray

Be gracious to your people, we entreat you, O Lord that they, repenting day by day of the things that displease you, may be more and more filled with love of you and of your commandments; and, being supported by your grace in this life, may come to the full enjoyment of eternal life in your everlasting kingdom; through Jesus Christ our Lord, who lives and reigns with you and the Holy Spirit, one God, for ever and ever. Amen.
—Lesser Feasts and Fasts

Reflect

The idea of a higher power—of God—is integral to the practice of yoga. In pure yoga fashion, yoga doesn't define God or prescribe a specific faith. Yoga invites us to devotion and provides a full set of tools and practices to help us. Everything you have learned in this book—the *yamas*, the *niyamas*, and *asana*—are tools to help you practice this final *niyama*, surrender and devotion to God.

How do we "do" devotion? What does it look like? Do we enter convents and monasteries? Do we retreat to ashrams on mountaintops? Do we pray eight times a day like the Benedictine monks and nuns?

Your devotion will take the form that God is calling you to. What matters is the desire to turn to God, or as Sharath Jois writes in *Astanga Yoga Anusthana* that we think of God as much as possible during our days.

Isvara pranidhana (devotion to God) is the end goal of yoga. We began with the premise that yoga is not a form of exercise but rather a spiritual practice. Yoga is about striving to attain spiritual knowledge, and then craving more so that ultimately you make spirituality the center of your life.

Spirituality does not have to be quiet and still, as some might expect. This is good news for many of us who have a hard time holding still! Yoga *asana* was devised as a moving prayer—a series of motions designed to draw our awareness inward. Yoga is movement that leads to stillness. And at the heart of that stillness, we find God.

Practice

Today, take notice of how your movements are like body prayer. Consider specifically the last posture, *savasana* or corpse pose. In that still moment of the practice, we are able to leave self-exploration behind and are finally quiet enough to explore God instead. Illusions melt away, and God is present in a way that is hard to know without the work of the postures, breath, and the *yamas* and *niyamas*. It is a stillness of the soul and a meeting of the Divine.

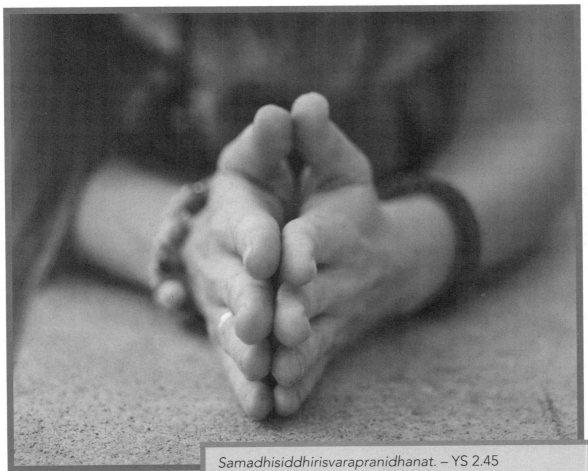

Samadhisiddhirisvarapranidhanat. – YS 2.45
By surrendering to God, we attain enlightenment.

Pray

> *Almighty God, through the incarnate Word you have caused us to be born anew of an imperishable and eternal seed: Look with compassion upon those who are being prepared for Holy Baptism, and grant that they may be built as living stones into a spiritual temple acceptable to you; through Jesus Christ our Lord, who lives and reigns with you and the Holy Spirit, one God, for ever and ever.* Amen. *—Lesser Feasts and Fasts*

Reflect

As we continue our exploration of *isvara pranidhana*, let us hear the words of Jesus. In John 5:30, Jesus describes his relationship to God by saying, "I can do nothing on my own. As I hear, I judge; and my judgment is just, because I do not seek my own will but the will of him who sent me."

Jesus shows his disciples (and us) the true nature of devotion to God. He surrenders to God's authority by stating that God controls all of creation, including our own desires. But instead of surrender creating a weak-willed follower, Jesus says that our devotion to God, our *isvara*, helps us know the will of God!

We stop seeking our own wants and selfish concerns and instead focus our energies on God's wants and desires. This is true for us on our mats and in the world. There may be days that we do not want to practice. There may be days when we do not feel inspired or close to God at all. There may be moments when we are tempted to leave behind our obligations as people of faith.

But those actions, feelings, or impulses do not reflect our true or best self. Following God in those difficult moments is part of a life of faith and devotion. Through our baptism, we have been given the power of the Holy Spirit to help us be faithful, even in those times of rebellion.

In our baptisms, we are told that the "bond that is established between God and ourselves is indissoluble." Nothing can break it. This is good news! It seems through sin and self wants, we always find new ways to distance ourselves from God. Yet, God is faithful, slow to anger and full of mercy.

Practice

On your mat today, spend time in thanksgiving for God who is with us no matter what, who loves us and is devoted to us. Let your practice today be an expression of gratitude for this kind of love. With every pose, find a way to rejoice—even during a pose that you hate the most! In this way, you show your love and devotion to the Spirit.

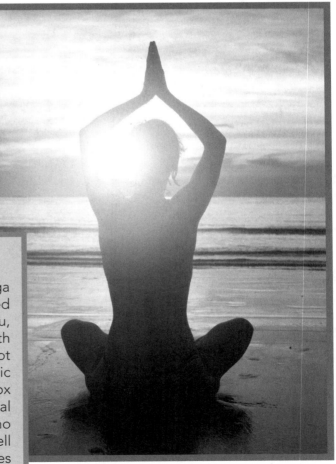

Is Yoga a Religion?

It is a common misconception that yoga is a Hindu practice. Yoga was developed in a country that is predominately Hindu, so many of its postures share names with Hindu gods and sages. But yoga is not Hindu. Yoga assumes God, but (in classic yoga fashion) does not put God in the box of a particular religion. Yoga is a spiritual tool that works equally well for people who practice any of the major world faiths as well as for people who categorize themselves as "spiritual but not religious."

Day 30
Isvara Pranidhana/Devotion to God

Pray

Almighty God our heavenly Father, renew in us the gifts of your mercy; increase our faith, strengthen our hope, enlighten our understanding, widen our charity, and make us ready to serve you; through Jesus Christ our Lord, who lives and reigns with you and the Holy Spirit, one God, for ever and ever. Amen.
—*Lesser Feasts and Fasts*

Reflect

You have been on a tremendous journey with God over these last few weeks. Every time you climbed onto your mat or considered how to live differently off the mat, you have encountered the Holy Spirit. In this last exercise, take time to reflect over each day and over the month-long journey. Write down three key learnings that you will take with you into the future. How has your life changed in big or small ways?

_____

_____

_____

_____

_____

_____

_____

_____

_____

_____

_____

Practice

This yogic journey has offered many suggestions on ways to increase *isvara pranidhana*. Yet there is no limit to the ways in which we can grow in our love and worship of God. Here are a few practices to help make devotion to God an everyday reality:

- Set aside time for prayer every day. It can be as little as five minutes as long as the practice is consistent and the time is truly set aside for God and God alone.
- Consider fasting once a month or week as a way to stay present in God's goodness. Every time you feel hunger, you will be reminded to say a prayer of thanksgiving for all the times you have been fed in so many ways.
- Read your Bible daily. This is the fount of God's goodness and message.
- Attend worship regularly. It is important to seek union with other followers to help you see God in community.
- Practice your yoga as often as you can. A little bit of yoga a lot is better than a lot of yoga a little. This is not only true for our bodies but also for our souls as well.
- Explore your own experiences with devotion in your journal.

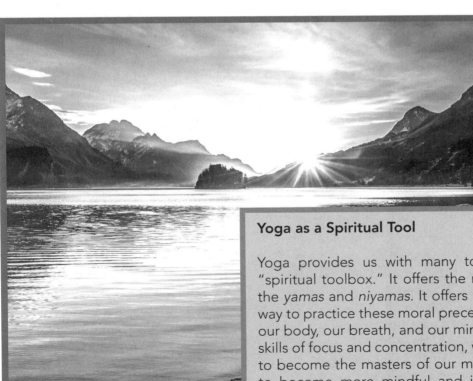

Yoga as a Spiritual Tool

Yoga provides us with many tools to put in our "spiritual toolbox." It offers the moral guidelines of the *yamas* and *niyamas*. It offers a safe and practical way to practice these moral precepts as we work with our body, our breath, and our mind. It teaches us the skills of focus and concentration, which help us begin to become the masters of our minds. Yoga helps us to become more mindful and intentional in all of our words, deeds, and even thoughts. Perhaps most powerfully, yoga reveals the interconnected nature of the world, reminding us again and again that we are valuable, unique pieces of the impossibly complex whole of creation.

Afterword

There is a long-standing tradition of holy pilgrimage in Christianity. For centuries, Christians have sought out sacred sites, places, and people and spent vast quantities of time and energy to get there. They came seeking not just the destination but the transformation that came with the journey itself. Sometimes these voyages were hazardous and difficult. Yet, each step a pilgrim took was viewed as an opportunity to walk toward God.

You too have been on a pilgrimage during these past thirty days. This pilgrimage may not have physically taken you off your mat, but you have nonetheless made a journey into a deeper relationship with God, yourself, and the world around you. And the beauty of this journey is that it is only beginning. There will never be an end to the lessons and strength that you can gain from a consistent practice of prayer and yoga. We hope this thirty-day journey has been enriching and will be part of the foundation for lifelong transformation.

May God's peace be with you.

Namaste.

Appendix

Glossary

Abhyasa: Sanskrit meaning practice. Pronounced ahb-high-ah-sa

Ahimsa: Sanskrit name for the first *yama*, nonviolence. Pronounced ah-heem-sa

Aparigraha: Sanskrit name for the fifth and final *yama*, non-possessiveness. Pronounced ah-par-ee-gra-ha

Asana: Sanskrit meaning yoga posture. Pronounced ah'-sa-na

Ashtanga: a particular branch or "kind" of yoga practiced by the authors. It was created by Sri K. Pattabhi Jois in Mysore, India. The current head teacher of the school (KPJAYI) is Jois's grandson, Sharath Jois. Pronouced ahsh-Than-ga

Asteya: Sanskrit name for the third *yama*, non-stealing. Pronounced: ah-stay-ya

Beginner's Mind: A state of mind or perspective where one approaches everything as if for the first time. This state of mind avoids assumptions and helps maintain an open sense of curiosity.

Bramacarya: Sanskrit name for the fourth *yama*, moderation or temperance. Pronounced: bra-ma-car-ya

Dandasana: Sanskrit name for a yoga posture called staff pose. Pronounced dahn-dah'-sa-na

Drishti: A gaze point in a yoga posture, for example, the tip of your nose or your finger tips, which adds another layer of focus to the practice. In balancing postures, your *drishti* can help also stabilize you. Pronounced drish'-tee

Isvara pranidhana: Sanskrit name for the fifth and final *niyama*, surrender or devotion to God. Pronounced ees'-vah-ra-pra-need-ha-na

Janu Sirsasana: Sanskrit name for a yoga posture called head to knee pose or seated tree pose. Pronounced ja-noo sheer-shas'-ah-na

Mantra: a word or phrase that is repeated internally in certain forms of meditation. Pronounced mahn-tra

Marichyasana: Sanskrit name for a yoga posture called seated twist. Pronounced mar-ee'-chee-as'-ah-na

Namaste: Sanskrit greeting that means "The light/good/divine in me recognizes and honors the same in you." Pronounced nah-ma-stay

Niyama: Sanskrit referring to five ethical practices designed to support us as we strive to live a spiritual life. They are commitments we make to ourselves. Pronouced nee-ya-ma

Om: This sound is often chanted in yoga classes and is said to be the sound of the vibration of the universe that we could hear if everything else were silent. Pronounced aum

Padangusthasana: Sanskrit name for a yoga posture called hand to big toe pose. Pronounced pa-dahn-goose-tha'-sa-na

Padmasana: Sanskrit name for a yoga posture called lotus pose. Pronounced Pahd-ma'-sa-na

Parsvakonasana: Sanskrit name for a yoga posture called extended side angle. Pronounced parse-vah-koe'-nah-sa-na

Posture: A yoga position or stretch. Sometimes referred to as a pose.

Practice: In yoga and in faith, this is the act of showing up, trying, sometimes succeeding and sometimes failing, but always knowing that showing up is enough.

Pranayama: Sanskrit for mindful breathing. There are many breathing exercises in yoga including alternate nostril breathing and bellows breath. Pronounced pra-na-ya'-ma

Prasarita padottanasana: Sanskrit name for a yoga posture call wide-legged forward fold. Pronounced pra-sah-ree'-ta pad-ah-ta'-nas-ah-na

Samadhi: The end goal of yoga, often referred to as enlightenment or spiritual liberation. Pronounced sah-mahd-hee'

Sanskrit: An ancient language of India. The language in which the original yoga scriptures, including Patañjali's *Yoga Sūtras* referenced in this book, were written.

Santosa: Sanskrit name for the second *niyama*, contentment. Pronounced san-toe-sa

Satya: Sanskrit name for the second *yama*, truthfulness. Pronounced saht-ya

Sauca: Sanskrit name for the first *niyama*, cleanliness or purity. Pronounced sow-ka

Savasana: Sanskrit name for a yoga posture called corpse or resting pose. Pronounced shah-vas'-ah-na

Setu bandasana: Sanskrit name for a yoga posture called bridge pose. Pronounced set-too bahn-das'-ah-na

Surya namaskar: Sanskrit name for a series or group of yoga postures called a sun salutation. Pronounced soor-ya nah'-ma-skar

Svadhyaya: Sanskrit name for the fourth *niyama*, self-study. Pronounced svad-high-ya

Tapas: Sanskrit meaning energy, zeal, passion, and commitment for whatever you have chosen to do. It is also the Sanskrit name for the third *niyama*, often referred to as self-discipline or zeal. Pronounced tah-pas

Trikonasana: Sanskrit name for triangle pose. Pronounced tree-koh-na'-sa-na

Vairaga: Sanskrit meaning renunciation. Pronounced vay-rah-ga

Vinyasa: A particular branch of yoga. In the *ashtanga* system, it refers to a series of movements between postures. Pronounced veen-ya-sa

Viparita karani: Sanskrit name for a yoga posture called legs up the wall pose. Pronounced vee-pa-rita ka-rah-nee

Virabhadrasana: Sanskrit name for a yoga posture called warrior pose. Pronounced veer-a-bah-drah-sa-na

Vrkasana: Sanskrit name for a yoga posture called tree pose. Pronounced vri-kah-sa-na

Yama: Sanskrit referring to five ethical practices designed to keep us in right relationship with ourselves, others and God. These are the foundation of a spiritually focused life. Pronouced ya-ma

Yoga: Sanskrit word meaning "to yoke." In a yoga practice we are yoking mind, body and spirit, allowing us to live more fully. In yoga philosophy, we are learning to yoke or manage the mind so that we are able to choose where we are focused at each moment of our days.

We encourage you to use this book at any point in the year. However, several times within the church's calendar offer poignant moments to take on a spiritual practice; this is especially true in the preparatory seasons of Advent and Lent. This section includes descriptions of the seasons as well as additional exercises to help you dive into the unique theological and experiential themes of these seasons.

Advent

Advent is a deep and holy time of waiting—waiting for the Messiah and preparing our hearts to greet him. This four-week season kicks off the new year for the church. The name itself comes from a Latin word meaning coming. During Advent, we prepare for the celebration of Christ's nativity as we look toward the future and the final coming of Christ in power and great glory.

Since Advent is a month long, the current meditations will work well as they are. However, we offer some additional practices that you and/or your group might add to your spiritual practice of prayer and yoga. These can deepen the seasonal themes of light, waiting, and joy.

- Advent Wreath: One of the most beautiful traditions of Advent is the weekly lighting of an Advent wreath. Traditionally made of fresh greens, an Advent wreath often has four candles, which represent the Sundays in each week of the season. Typically, these candles are blue or purple. Additionally, a white candle is used in the center and is known as the Christ candle. It is lit on Christmas Eve and should burn for the twelve days of Christmas. Feel free to get creative with your Advent wreath. For example, just use candles if finding greens is an issue. The lighting of a candle before starting your practice is a lovely way to make the time on your mat holy and sacred.
- Advent Spiral: An Advent spiral is a large spiral path that is spread out on the floor so people can walk through it. This spiral—a labyrinth of sorts—offers a simple way to celebrate the mood of the season, of moving from darkness to light. In the center of the spiral we find the Holy Family as we join with them in their journey toward Bethlehem. People walk the unlit path, one at a time, into the center of the spiral path of evergreens, carrying their candle. They light their candle and carefully place it down along the path as they return. Place yoga mats on the outside of the spiral to practice around this holy light.

- Begin the new year of the church by committing to praying for a person for a season or every single day for a year using the Daily Office. Try using the website: www.prayer.forwardmovement.org. Saying a prayer at the start or conclusion of your practice can turn that time into dedication and petition for your loved one.

Lent

Like Advent, Lent is a time of preparation as we move toward the great feast of Easter. Since the early church, Christians have marked this season with prayer, penitence, fasting, self-denial, and acts of charity. As you have seen in this book, these themes are often explored in yoga as well, as both practices call us into fuller relationship with Christ.

In the Western church, the forty days of Lent extend from Ash Wednesday through Holy Saturday, omitting Sundays. The last three days of Lent are the sacred Triduum of Maundy Thursday, Good Friday, and Holy Saturday. Today Lent has reacquired its significance as the final preparation of adult candidates for baptism.

Faith with a Twist offers thirty days of prayer, reflection, and practice. If you want to adapt your practice for the season of Lent, you can extend it to the full season by adding Sundays as well as Holy Week to your journey. We have prepared a free downloadable resource that follows the same format of pray, reflect, practice. It is available on the *Faith with a Twist* product page on the Forward Movement website, www.forwardmovement.org.

Easter

Easter is the most important time in the life of the church year! This is a fifty-day season celebrating the resurrection of Jesus and the call to new life that it offers. Here are some ways that you can celebrate Easter by extending your practice beyond the thirty days found in this book:

- **Days 31-38: Meditation**
  Add a longer time of meditation to your daily asana practice. In particular, spend an extended time in *savasana* or corpse pose. This restorative posture comes at the end of every yoga practice to symbolize the death of a practice. When you come out of it, a new world of possibilities awaits you. This mirrors the call to resurrected life that we are given in Easter—we die to our old way of sin so that we might live a new life with Christ.

- **Days 39-46: *Seva***
  Delve into the yogic concept of *seva*, which means "selfless service." This concept invites us to share the peace and joy that we have found in our faith and practice and pass it on to others. There is never a better time

to express our gratitude for the love we have been given than during the Easter season. Choose one of these activities or one of your own each day this week.

- Volunteer at a local soup kitchen.
- Commit to praying for a person for a season or every single day for a year using the Daily Office. Try using the website: www.prayer.forwardmovement.org.
- Commit to praying for friends and family members on special anniversaries and dates such as their birthday, their baptismal anniversary, or the feast of the saint who shares their name.
- Hold an "energy fast" where you do not use any electronics and use the time to reconnect with your family.
- Adopt a new ecofriendly habit (such as composting, committing to reducing your carbon footprint, or riding a bike to work) as a gift to the planet, yourself, your (future) children, or (future) grandchildren.
- Start a garden or plant a tree.
- Using the website www.theuniformproject.com/#!diy, take the uniform challenge. Wear the same 1-6 pieces of clothing for a long period of time (a week, month, year) to save money on disposable fashion and raise money and awareness for a cause. You will be amazed by how many different ways you can wear just one article of clothing!
- Write a letter to someone who is far away, elderly, or very young.
- Write a letter to your politicians to help this and future generations.
- Take over a chore or responsibility for someone else. Or, take over a duty (such as yard work or shopping) for someone who can no longer manage those tasks.
- Learn a new skill or craft such as knitting or painting and create gifts with meaning.
- Spend quality time with someone.

- **Day 47: Take Your Practice Further**
Commit to taking your yoga practice further by finding a teacher or a class. Look for someone who seeks to incorporate the prayerful aspect of yoga as well as the *asana* to keep your journey of inner peace going.

- **Days 48-50: Get Involved!**
If you do not already have a worshiping community, visit a local church to learn about the community, spiritual life, worship, and outreach opportunities. You can find a local Episcopal church here: www.episcopalchurch.org/find-a-church. If you are a member of a church, visit it today and offer to do something to help.

Resources

For video of yoga practices and additional resources, visit www.thehiveapiary.com

Astanga Yoga Anusthana by Jois. R. Sharath (KPJAYI Mysore, 2013)

Ashtanga Yoga: The Practice Manual by David Swenson (Ashtanga Yoga Productions, 1999)

The Breath of God: An Approach to Prayer by Nancy Roth (Cowley Publications, 1990)

Living Your Yoga: Finding the Spiritual in Everyday Life by Judith Lasater (Rodmell Press, 2000)

Meditations from the Mat by Rolf Gates (Anchor Books, 2002)

Slim, Calm, Sexy Yoga, "Relaxation," by Tara Stiles (Rodale, 2010)

The Yoga Sutra of Patanjali: A New Translation with Commentary by Chip Hartranft (Shambhala Classics, 2003)